# The
# Twelve Steps
# *and*
# Twelve Traditions
# *of*
# Overeaters Anonymous

## Second Edition

The Twelve Steps and Twelve Traditions of Overeaters Anonymous

Overeaters Anonymous, Inc.

World Service Office

PO Box 44020, Rio Rancho NM 87174-4020 USA

1-505-891-2664

www.oa.org

Printed in the United States of America.

Library of Congress Catalog Card No.: 2017917353

ISBN: 978-1-889681-20-7

# PREAMBLE

Overeaters Anonymous is a Fellowship of individuals who, through shared experience, strength, and hope, are recovering from compulsive overeating. We welcome everyone who wants to stop eating compulsively. There are no dues or fees for members; we are self-supporting through our own contributions, neither soliciting nor accepting outside donations. OA is not affiliated with any public or private organization, political movement, ideology, or religious doctrine; we take no position on outside issues. Our primary purpose is to abstain from compulsive eating and compulsive food behaviors and to carry the message of recovery through the Twelve Steps of OA to those who still suffer.

# CONTENTS

**Introduction to the Twelve Steps** . . . . . . . . . . . . . . . . . . . . . . . 1
Step One . . . . . . . . . . . . . . . . . . . . . . . . . . . . . . . . . . . . . . . . . 3
Step Two . . . . . . . . . . . . . . . . . . . . . . . . . . . . . . . . . . . . . . . . . 9
Step Three . . . . . . . . . . . . . . . . . . . . . . . . . . . . . . . . . . . . . . 17
Step Four . . . . . . . . . . . . . . . . . . . . . . . . . . . . . . . . . . . . . . . 25
Step Five . . . . . . . . . . . . . . . . . . . . . . . . . . . . . . . . . . . . . . . 39
Step Six . . . . . . . . . . . . . . . . . . . . . . . . . . . . . . . . . . . . . . . . 45
Step Seven . . . . . . . . . . . . . . . . . . . . . . . . . . . . . . . . . . . . . . 51
Step Eight . . . . . . . . . . . . . . . . . . . . . . . . . . . . . . . . . . . . . . 57
Step Nine . . . . . . . . . . . . . . . . . . . . . . . . . . . . . . . . . . . . . . . 63
Step Ten . . . . . . . . . . . . . . . . . . . . . . . . . . . . . . . . . . . . . . . . 69
Step Eleven . . . . . . . . . . . . . . . . . . . . . . . . . . . . . . . . . . . . . 75
Step Twelve . . . . . . . . . . . . . . . . . . . . . . . . . . . . . . . . . . . . . 81

**Introduction to the Twelve Traditions** . . . . . . . . . . . . . . . . . 89
Tradition One . . . . . . . . . . . . . . . . . . . . . . . . . . . . . . . . . . . . 91
Tradition Two . . . . . . . . . . . . . . . . . . . . . . . . . . . . . . . . . . . . 99
Tradition Three . . . . . . . . . . . . . . . . . . . . . . . . . . . . . . . . . 107
Tradition Four . . . . . . . . . . . . . . . . . . . . . . . . . . . . . . . . . . 113
Tradition Five . . . . . . . . . . . . . . . . . . . . . . . . . . . . . . . . . . 119
Tradition Six . . . . . . . . . . . . . . . . . . . . . . . . . . . . . . . . . . . 125
Tradition Seven . . . . . . . . . . . . . . . . . . . . . . . . . . . . . . . . . 131
Tradition Eight . . . . . . . . . . . . . . . . . . . . . . . . . . . . . . . . . 139
Tradition Nine . . . . . . . . . . . . . . . . . . . . . . . . . . . . . . . . . . 145
Tradition Ten . . . . . . . . . . . . . . . . . . . . . . . . . . . . . . . . . . . 151
Tradition Eleven . . . . . . . . . . . . . . . . . . . . . . . . . . . . . . . . 157
Tradition Twelve . . . . . . . . . . . . . . . . . . . . . . . . . . . . . . . . 163

The Twelve Steps of Overeaters Anonymous . . . . . . . . . . . . . . 169
The Twelve Traditions of Overeaters Anonymous . . . . . . . . . 170
Index . . . . . . . . . . . . . . . . . . . . . . . . . . . . . . . . . . . . . . . . . . 172

# INTRODUCTION TO
# THE TWELVE STEPS

We of Overeaters Anonymous have found in this Fellowship a way to recover from the disease of compulsive overeating. We use "compulsive overeating" and "compulsive eating" interchangeably. These terms include, but are not limited to, overeating, under-eating, food addiction, anorexia, bulimia, binge eating, over-exercising, purging, and other compulsive food behaviors. No matter what form our disease takes, anyone having a problem with food can find help in Overeaters Anonymous. After repeated failures to control our eating and our weight, we now have a solution that works. Our solution is a program of recovery—a program of Twelve simple Steps. By following these Steps, thousands of OA members have stopped eating compulsively.

In OA we have no program of diets and exercise, no scales, no magic pills. What we do have to offer is far greater than any of these things—a Fellowship in which we find and share the healing power of love. Our common bonds are two: the disease of compulsive eating from which we all have suffered, and the solution that we all are finding as we live by the Principles embodied in these Steps. Since our program is based on the Twelve Steps, we would like to offer here a study of those Steps, sharing how we follow them to recover from compulsive eating. We hope in this way to provide help for those who still suffer from our disease.

If you think you may be a compulsive eater, give yourself a chance for recovery by trying the OA program. Our way of life, based on the Twelve Steps and Twelve Traditions, has brought us physical, emotional, and spiritual healing that we don't hesitate to call miraculous. What works for us will work for you too.

# STEP ONE

We admitted we were powerless over food—
that our lives had become unmanageable.

---

*SPIRITUAL PRINCIPLE*

## HONESTY

In Overeaters Anonymous we begin our program of recovery by admitting that we're powerless over food. Some of us have difficulty with this admission because we've had so much experience in trying to control our eating. At one time, or periodically, most of us were able to do so. Our eating may be out of control right now, we persisted in thinking, but someday soon we'll again find the strength of character needed to limit our eating excesses, and this time we'll keep them under control. For all of us, however, the days of controlled eating grew fewer and farther apart, until at last we came to OA, looking for a new solution.

In OA we learn that a lack of willpower isn't what makes us compulsive eaters. In fact, compulsive overeaters often exhibit an exceptional amount of willpower. But compulsive eating is an illness that cannot be controlled by willpower. None of us decided to have this disorder, any more than we would have decided to have any other disease. We can now cease blaming ourselves or others for our compulsive overeating.

The disease of compulsive eating is threefold in nature: physical, emotional, and spiritual. Compulsive eating does not stem simply from bad eating habits learned in childhood, nor just from adjustment problems, nor merely from a love of food, though all three of these may be factors in its development. It may be that many of us were born with a physical or emotional predisposition to eat compulsively. Whatever the cause, today we are not like normal people when it comes to food and eating behaviors.

Like compulsive overeaters, normal eaters sometimes find pleasure and escape from life's problems in excess food. A normal eater, however, gets full and loses interest in food. Compulsive eaters often have an abnormal reaction to food. Some of us overindulge and can't quit, and then we crave more. Sometimes the craving is for a particular food; we feel compelled to eat another serving after we've finished the first … and then another … and another. Other compulsive eaters indulge in the illusion of control through restricting food intake. Some of us purge after eating in an effort to control our weight. What all compulsive eaters have in common is that our bodies and minds seem to send us signals about food that are quite different from those the normal eater receives. We have found through much experience that, no matter how long we abstain from eating compulsively and no matter how adept we become at facing life, we will always have these abnormal tendencies. Those of us who have returned to our former compulsive eating behaviors, even after years in recovery, have found it harder than ever to stop.

Clearly, if we are to live free of the bondage of compulsive eating, we must abstain from all foods and eating behaviors that cause us to eat compulsively. But this, too, has proven impossible for us to do by our willpower alone. Before we found OA, every diet or period of control was followed by a period of uncontrolled eating.

This is because our malady was not just physical in nature; it was emotional and spiritual as well. We were obsessed with food, and no amount of self-control or weight loss could cure us. Because of this obsession, the day always came when the excess food looked so inviting to us we couldn't resist, and our firm resolutions were forgotten. Sooner or later, we lost control and returned to compulsive eating and compulsive food behaviors.

This mental obsession was something we couldn't be rid of by our unaided human will. If we were to stop eating compulsively, and stay stopped, we had to find another power, stronger than ourselves, for relief.

Most of us have tried to deny to ourselves that we have this disease. In OA we are encouraged to take a good look at our compulsive eating, obesity, obsession with food, and body image and the self-destructive things we have done to avoid obesity—the dieting, starving, over-exercising, or purging. Once we honestly examine our histories, we can deny it no longer: Our eating and our attitudes toward food are not normal; we have this disease.

Part two of Step One, admitting "that our lives had become unmanageable," has also been difficult for many of us. We felt that we had managed very well in life, despite our problems with food and weight. Many of us held responsible jobs and ran our households with reasonable success. We had friends who liked us, and many of us had fairly good marriages. That these didn't make us happy was surely due to the fact that we were fat (or felt we were). If we could just get to the perfect weight, life would be wonderful. Surely it would be exaggerating to say we were incapable of managing our lives. We certainly could use some help with the compulsive eating, but with the rest of life, we were doing fine.

Again, an honest look at our lives helped us to take Step One. Were we really excelling at our jobs, or just getting by? Were our homes pleasant places to be, or had we been living in an atmosphere of depression or anger? Had our chronic unhappiness over our eating problems affected our relationships? Were we truly in touch with our feelings, or had we buried our anger and fear in false cheerfulness?

We sometimes recognized we had problems, but felt that life would be manageable if only we could stop the compulsive eating. Whenever we did stop, however, we found life unbearable. Even getting to our desired weight didn't cure our unhappiness.

Many of us believed that our lives would be manageable if only others around us would do as we wanted. We thought everything would be fine if only our bosses would recognize our worth, if only our spouses would give us the attention we needed, if only our children were well-behaved, if only our parents would leave us alone. Our lives became unmanageable when the car wouldn't start, the computer broke down, or our bank account wouldn't balance. We suffered from other people's unmanaged lives or from bad luck. What alternative did we have? We ate to sate the fears, the anxieties, the angers, the disappointments. We ate to escape the pressures of our problems or the boredom of everyday life. We procrastinated, we hid, and we ate.

Before we came to OA and began discussing our experiences honestly with other compulsive overeaters, we didn't realize how much we had damaged ourselves and others by attempting to manage every detail of life. It was only after we began to recover that we saw the childish self-centeredness of our willful actions. By trying to control others through manipulation and direct force, we had hurt our loved ones. When we tried to control ourselves, we wound up demoralized. Even when we succeeded, it wasn't enough to make us happy. We hid from our pain by eating compulsively, so we didn't learn from our mistakes; we never grew up.

Some of us resisted Step One because it seemed like negative thinking. If we tell ourselves we're powerless over food, we reasoned, then we program ourselves to go right on eating compulsively!

Later we discovered that, far from being a negative factor, the admission of our powerlessness over food has opened the door to an amazing newfound power. For the first time in our lives, we recognized, acknowledged, and accepted the truth about ourselves. We *are* compulsive eaters. We *do* have an incurable disease. Diabetics who need to be on insulin risk blindness and possible death unless they recognize the truth of their diabetic condition, accept it, and take the prescribed medication. So it is with compulsive overeaters. As long as we refuse to recognize that we have this debilitating, progressive, and ultimately fatal disease, we are not motivated to get the daily treatment that brings about our recovery. Denial of the truth leads to destruction. Only an honest admission to ourselves of the reality of our condition can save us from our destructive eating.

The same principle applies to our unmanageable lives. As long as we believe that we already know what is best for us, we cling to our habitual ways of thinking and acting. Yet these ways of thinking and acting got us into the unhealthy, unhappy condition we were in when we came to OA. In Step One, we acknowledge this truth about ourselves: Our current methods of managing have not been successful, and we need to find a new approach to life. Having acknowledged this truth, we are free to change and to learn.

Once we have become teachable, we can give up old thought and behavior patterns that have failed us in the past, beginning with our attempts to control our eating and our weight. Honest appraisal of our experience has convinced us that we can't handle life through self-will alone. First we grasp this knowledge intellectually, and then finally, we come to believe it in our hearts. When this happens, we have taken the First Step and are ready to move ahead in our program of recovery.

# STEP TWO

Came to believe that a Power greater than ourselves
could restore us to sanity.

---

*SPIRITUAL PRINCIPLE*

**HOPE**

Many of us compulsive overeaters tend to look at this Step and say: "Restore me to sanity? I don't need that. I'm perfectly sane. I just have an eating problem." But how sane are we, really?

When we look with complete honesty at our lives, we see that where eating is concerned we have acted in an extremely irrational and self-destructive manner. Under the compulsion to overeat, many of us have done things no sane person would think of doing. We have driven miles in the dead of night to satisfy a craving for food. We have eaten food that was frozen, burnt, stale, or even dangerously spoiled. We have eaten food off other people's plates, off the floor, and off the ground. We have dug food out of the garbage and eaten it.

We have frequently lied about what we have eaten—lied to ourselves and to others because we didn't want to face the truth about what we do when it comes to food. We have stolen food from our friends, family, and employers, as well as from the grocery store. We have also stolen money to buy food. We have eaten beyond the point of being full, beyond the point of being sick of eating. We have continued to overeat, knowing all the while we were disfiguring and maiming our bodies. We have isolated ourselves to eat, damaging our relationships and denying ourselves full social lives. Because of our compulsive eating, we have turned ourselves into objects of ridicule and we have destroyed our health.

Then, horrified by what we were doing to ourselves with food, we became obsessed with diets. We spent lots of money on weight-loss schemes; we bought all sorts of appetite suppressants; we joined diet clubs and fitness centers; we had ourselves hypnotized and analyzed; we had major surgery on our digestive systems; we had our ears stapled or our jaws wired shut. All of this we did willingly, hoping we could still eat all we wanted and be free of the compulsion.

Some of us went from doctor to doctor looking for a cure. The doctors gave us diets, but we had no better success with those than with the other diets we'd been on. The doctors prescribed shots and pills. Those worked for a while, but we inevitably lost control and overate again, putting back on the weight we had worked so hard to lose and frequently gaining more.

Many of us tried fasting, with and without a doctor's supervision. Usually we lost weight, but as soon as we started eating again, the compulsive eating behavior returned, along with the weight. Some of us learned to purge ourselves with vomiting, laxatives, or excessive exercise. We damaged our digestive systems and our teeth while we starved our bodies of the nutrients we needed to live. Some of us were so terrified of gaining weight, we went to great lengths to restrict what we ate. We refused to eat certain foods, we developed complex rituals around food, and we tried to avoid eating whenever possible. Other people told us we were too thin, but we thought they were overreacting. Our weight went down, sometimes to dangerous levels, but we still felt fat.

Most of us got plenty of advice from others about how to get to our "ideal" size, but nothing permanently solved our problem. We found that no matter what we did to ease our turmoil, our compulsive eating behavior eventually returned. Over time, we became weary and discouraged from battling with weight, and our self-esteem went down. Still, we could never accept our powerlessness. The prospect of being obsessed with food and weight, sick, and out of control for the rest of our lives led some of us to conclude that life was simply not worth living. Many of us thought about suicide. Some of us tried it.

Most of us, however, never reached suicidal desperation. Instead, we took comfort in a feeling that everything was all right as long as we got enough to eat. The only trouble was that, as our compulsive eating progressed, we ate more and more, yet we were never satisfied. Instead of bringing comfort, the overeating backfired. The more we ate, the more we suffered, yet we continued to overeat. Our true insanity could be seen in the fact that we kept right on trying to find comfort in excess food, long after it began to cause us misery.

Once we honestly looked at our lives, it became easy for us to admit we had acted insanely where food and weight were concerned. Many of us, however, were able to confine our compulsive overeating to the hours when we were alone and to carry on with relatively normal lives. We worked hard during the day and ate hard at night. Surely we were sane in most respects.

More self-examination revealed many areas in which our lives were out of balance. We had to admit that we had not acted sanely when we responded to our children's needs for attention by yelling at them, or when we were jealously possessive of our mates. Too much of the time we had lived in fear and anxiety. More comfortable with food than with people, we sometimes limited our social lives. We closed the curtains, stopped answering the phone, and hid in the house.

When we were around other people, we smiled and agreed when we really wanted to say no. Some of us were unable to stand up for ourselves in abusive relationships; we felt we deserved the abuse. Or, we focused on others' faults and thought for hours about what they should do to solve their problems, while our own problems went unsolved.

Compulsive eaters are often people of extremes. We overreacted to slight provocations while ignoring the real issues in our lives. We were obsessively busy, then we were exhausted and unable to act. We were wildly excited then deeply depressed. We saw the whole world in black and white. If we couldn't have it all, we didn't want any; if we couldn't be the best, we didn't want to participate.

Little by little, we saw how much pain our way of living was causing us. Gradually, we came to believe we needed to change. In all of life, as well as with the food, we were irrational, unbalanced, and insane. If our willpower and determination couldn't change our unsuccessful way of living, what could? Clearly, if we were to be restored to sanity, we had to find a Power greater than ourselves. At this point, most of us had trouble for one reason or another with Step Two. Some of us did not believe in God. We despaired of finding a solution to our problems if that meant we had to "find God." Some of us walked out of our first meeting when we heard that three-letter word mentioned and didn't return until years of more compulsive eating had made us desperate. Those of us who stuck around and began working the Steps made a wonderful discovery. OA doesn't tell us we have to believe in God—only that "a Power greater than ourselves could restore us to sanity." We are invited to define that Power however we wish and relate to it in whatever way works for us. OA only suggests that we remain open to spiritual growth and show tolerance for others by neither criticizing nor promoting specific religious doctrines in OA meetings.

Ours is a spiritual program, not a religious one. We have no creeds or doctrines, only our own experiences of recovery. Atheists and agnostics are welcome in OA and have found recovery.

How have we who were not believers in God come to believe in a Higher Power?

It usually started as we sat in an OA meeting and experienced the camaraderie of our fellow compulsive overeaters. Here were people who understood us and cared about us. We could be totally honest about ourselves, and they still accepted us unconditionally. This acceptance grew into love, carrying with it a power that seemed to stay with us as we left our OA meetings. It was not too great a leap of faith to believe that this shared love was a Power greater than ourselves that could help lead us to sanity. The love of the group, then, became our Higher Power.

Before long, we usually asked other OA members to be our sponsors. Most of us chose someone with whom we felt a kinship or in whom we saw recovery. As we developed personal relationships with our sponsors, the love of the OA group came to us in a deeper way. Sponsors answered our questions, listened to our problems, shared our tears and laughter, and guided us in recovery as they helped us apply OA Principles in our lives. For the first time ever, we felt the relief of not having to face our problems alone. This relationship represented a Higher Power in which we could believe.

However, OA members are human. Sometimes, when our groups or sponsors failed us in some way, we felt cut off from the support that had come to mean so much to us, and our new sanity seemed threatened. We now needed a more reliable way of relating to a Higher Power. At this point, we learned we could "act as if." This didn't mean we were to be dishonestly pious or pretend we believed in God when we didn't. It meant we were free to set aside theological arguments and examine the idea of spiritual power in light of our own desperate need for help with our lives.

Some of us began by asking ourselves: "What do I need from a Higher Power? What would I like such a Power to be and do in my life?" Once we identified this Power for ourselves, we found we felt at ease with it. Then we began to act as if such a Power existed, and we found good things happening to us as a result. Little by little, as we experienced changes for the better in our lives, we came to believe in a Power greater than ourselves that could restore us to sanity.

Those of us who arrived at OA with a set of religious beliefs usually looked at this Step and said, "No problem. I'm beyond that Step.

I already believe in God." Then, to our dismay, some of us found ourselves having more trouble with the OA program than agnostics or atheists. Sometimes we had trouble because we believed in God's existence, but we didn't really believe God could and would deal with our compulsive eating. Perhaps we didn't believe that our compulsive eating was a spiritual problem, or we felt that God was concerned only with more important matters and expected us to control such a simple thing as our eating. We failed to understand that God loves us in our totality and is willing and able to help us in everything we do, that God will help us with every decision, even food choices and amounts.

Many of us had asked God to help us control our weight, and this prayer hadn't worked. Later we understood why our pleas for help seemed to fall on deaf ears. What we were really asking God to do was remove our fat while allowing us to go on eating whatever we wanted, whenever we wanted. Most of us also needed to learn to ask other people for help and to let God speak to us through our fellows. In OA, God's healing power comes to us through a caring community of other compulsive overeaters. Before we joined the OA Fellowship, our prayers for help might have gone unanswered simply because we were never meant to face this disease in isolation. We were meant to open up so that we might learn to receive love and to truly love others.

Whatever the case, after years of making vows and saying prayers but then eating compulsively again, we were left without faith that God could restore us to sanity about food. We believed intellectually that God could do anything, but deep in our hearts we "knew" God couldn't help us with this area of our lives. It was this negative concept about God we had to change if we were to find recovery. How could we do this? We became willing to start fresh with our Higher Power. Our heartfelt concept of God wasn't working, so we became willing for it to be changed. Just like atheists or agnostics, we could begin to do this by asking ourselves what, exactly, we needed and wanted God to be to us and to do for us. Then we acted as if God were really exactly what we wanted and needed our Higher Power to be. We became willing to let go of any concept about God that wasn't helping us to recover from compulsive eating. We had to replace our old ideas about God with a faith that works. This was both humbling and frightening for us, but once we became willing to do it, surprising things began to happen.

For all of us, coming to believe was something that happened as we began taking actions that others told us had worked for them. Whether we believed these actions would work for us didn't seem to matter. Once we took the action and saw it work, we began to believe. Then we tried other suggestions, and our lives began to be transformed.

This willingness to act on faith, then, was the key to Step Two. It was the beginning of the healing process and relief from the food compulsion. We began to see stability in our unbalanced lives. We responded to the love we had been shown in OA, by taking action and working the Steps. The result was a new faith in ourselves, in others, and in the power of that love. We had begun to develop a new relationship with a Power greater than ourselves, and we were ready to move ahead with our program of recovery.

# STEP THREE

Made a decision to turn our will and our lives over to
the care of God *as we understood Him.*

---

*SPIRITUAL PRINCIPLE*

### FAITH

It has been said that the first three Steps of the Overeaters
Anonymous program are simply "I can't; God can; I think I'll
let God!" In Step One we became convinced that we could manage
neither our eating nor our other problems by our own will alone.
In Step Two we added to this acceptance of our utter helplessness
a newfound faith that there exists a Power greater than us that can
relieve us of the obsession with food and restore us to sanity in all
areas of life.

It is impossible to take Step Three until we have taken the first
two Steps. Once we have fully acknowledged our fatal powerlessness and have come to believe that there is a solution, however, the
Third Step is simple. If we want to live free of the killing disease of

compulsive eating, we accept help without reservation from a Power greater than ourselves and begin taking the actions that will allow us to receive that help. We now say yes to this Power, deciding from here on to follow spiritual guidance in making every decision.

Note we have said this Step is simple; we have not said it is easy. It is not easy, because, for every one of us, this decision means we must now adopt a new and unfamiliar way of thinking and acting on life. From now on, we let go of our preconceived notions about what is right for us. When faced with choices, we earnestly seek guidance from our Higher Power, and when that guidance comes, we act on it. Our new way of life begins with a willingness to adopt a whole new attitude about weight control, body image, and eating. The OA Twelve Step program differs greatly from the diet and weight-loss programs we tried in the past. Those systems gave us diets to follow but made *us* responsible for adhering to them. In OA we are given no diets, but we are shown a program of recovery that addresses the emotional and spiritual nature of our problem in addition to the physical. Weight loss is not our only goal, and we accept that even a "perfect" body (if there were such a thing) would not make us happy. Our primary purpose is to abstain from compulsive eating and compulsive food behaviors. We know that in order to do so we need to work the remaining nine Steps of the program.

At one time or another, since we joined OA, most of us have experienced a period of complete freedom from the obsession with food and the compulsion to overeat. For many of us, this freedom came when we took Step Three and turned the entire problem over to our Higher Power. Suddenly we no longer thought much about food and eating. When mealtime came, we ate moderately, felt satisfied, and stopped eating. It was as if some miracle had given us a healthy attitude about food and eating.

For many of us, however, this reprieve didn't last forever. Gradually food regained its dominance in our thoughts. Eventually the day came when we again wanted food we didn't need, and staying away from eating compulsively became more difficult for us. Did this mean that we hadn't really taken Step Three after all? Sometimes that was the case, but usually it simply meant the OA honeymoon was over. What we needed now was a way of remaining abstinent and living sanely through good times and bad. Continuing to take the actions outlined in OA's Steps allows us to do that.

Often we caused ourselves problems because we didn't realize that there were some foods and eating behaviors we could handle comfortably and some we couldn't. Many members of OA have been able to identify certain foods and eating behaviors that lead us into compulsive eating. Acceptance of these facts about ourselves gives us hope. For we know that by simply eliminating these foods and eating behaviors from our lives we will experience fewer struggles with our disease. We are individuals with our own individual nutritional needs, and we've found that what is a healthy choice for some might be lethal for others. People who come to OA are sometimes confused by the lack of dietary regulations. "If OA doesn't give us any rules to follow," they ask, "how are we to find the guidance we must have to avoid compulsive eating?" The decision we have made in Step Three answers this important question. We have found that when we give up self-will regarding food and completely turn our lives over to our Higher Power, we receive all kinds of guidance.

For instance, after years spent in the struggle with this disease, we have been able to take an honest look at our past experiences and identify for ourselves the specific kinds of foods and eating behaviors that give us the most trouble. Some of us have been given eating restrictions by qualified professionals because of special physical problems or needs. Many of us know a lot about sound nutrition, but we have never before been able to put this knowledge into effect because our food obsession interfered. Now that we are working the Steps and accept our Higher Power's guidance, we have been given the power of choice about our eating. We find we are led to make better decisions about our food. It becomes more obvious to us which foods and behaviors are keeping us trapped in our disease. We find that, once we recognize our own particular problem areas, we become willing to select foods and behaviors that don't fuel our obsession.

When we are developing our plan of eating, many of us have been helped by discussing our particular problems with our sponsors and health professionals. Of course, the final responsibility for what we eat and don't eat rests with us, but we have found that getting honest about our food behaviors with another person can help us find our way.

The definition of abstinence has been refined over the years as the OA Fellowship has clarified the meaning of abstinence for all of our members. It is important to remember that abstinence is not the exact content of our plan of eating, which we are each responsible to determine and follow as we surrender to our Higher Power's guidance.

Nor is abstinence about what we weigh, although attaining and maintaining a healthy body weight is a result of our abstinence. Abstinence is refraining from compulsive eating and compulsive food behaviors that create the obsessive thinking about and destructive acting out with food.

A plan of eating helps us each day to get and remain abstinent. Food plans may change over time as our circumstances change or as we discover new or different foods or behaviors from which we must abstain.

All of this experience, knowledge, and help is augmented by a source of wisdom inside us that becomes more powerful as we recover from compulsive eating and develop our relationship with our Higher Power through prayer and meditation. This inner resource is our intuition. When we place our will and our lives in God's care in Step Three, we give God our intuition as well. Intuition is supposed to be God's direct line into our minds and hearts, but our problems and our self-will have interfered with this connection. As we work the Steps, the interference begins to be removed, and intuition begins to function properly, helping us to focus on God's will, both for our eating and for the living of our lives.

It is important to bear in mind that knowledge of ourselves and our nutritional needs is useless without the kind of help we find through working all of OA's Twelve Steps. Many of us have tried for years to find the perfect way of eating and stick to it. In order to continue being abstinent, we have to have a Power greater than ourselves operating in our lives daily. This is always available to us as long as we continue working the Twelve Steps and living out our decision to trust God's guidance in everything we do. As we become aware of what our healthy eating guidelines should be, we ask God for the willingness and the ability to live within them each day. We ask and we receive, first the willingness, and then the ability. We can count on this without fail.

As we continue abstaining, we find we can depend on God to eliminate our yearning for the kind of eating that harms us. Much of the time, we no longer want to eat unwisely and we come to prefer foods that are appropriate for us. This miracle of sanity, the result of working OA's Twelve Steps, is an everyday reality for thousands of recovering compulsive overeaters. We find we are seldom obsessed with eating and food, that it is possible for us to continue eating moderate, nutritious meals, one day at a time, day after day, month after month, year after year.

Do we ever achieve a permanent freedom from food obsession? Yes, and no. OA longtimers do have this miraculous freedom most days, but occasionally, for some, the obsession returns. How do we get through these times without returning to compulsive eating? We don't panic. Instead, we quietly reaffirm our personal guidelines and ask our Higher Power to help us continue living within them. Then we turn away from food and eating to focus our attention on our OA Fellowship and the Twelve Steps. As we work the Steps, using the Tools of the program—a plan of eating, sponsorship, meetings, telephone, writing, literature, action plan, anonymity, and service[1]— we find the help we need. OA friends lovingly remind us that "This too shall pass." It does pass, and our obsession is lifted again. This abstinent way of life continues on a daily basis so long as we con-

---

[1] The Tool "abstinence," listed in the first edition, was replaced by the Tool "a plan of eating" at the 1995 World Service Business Conference. Abstinence remains our primary purpose, as outlined in the OA Preamble. The Tool "action plan" was recognized at the 2011 World Service Business Conference.

tinue to trust a Higher Power with our lives, renew our Step Three commitment daily, and practice all of OA's Twelve Steps.

Inexperienced in this way of living, many of us have asked, "How do I reach this decision to turn my will and life over to a Higher Power? What exactly do I have to do?" It helps to understand that once we make this decision our approach to all choices will be like our approach to our food. We will no longer simply do what we feel like doing or what we think we can get away with. Instead, we will earnestly seek to learn God's will for us, then we will act accordingly. Working the Steps will help us to let go of fear and indecision. If we are sincere, our Higher Power will give us the knowledge of our best course in life, along with the willingness and ability to follow that course, even when it seems difficult and uncomfortable.

In learning God's will, we may again refer to our experience, knowledge, common sense, and intuition and to the wisdom of spiritual mentors. If something has repeatedly worked well for us or for someone else in a similar situation, we may assume it will work in our present situation, ultimately bringing good to us and to others, which is God's will. For instance, we might find from experience that when we're feeling unstable, going to OA meetings helps us to reconnect with other OA members and our Higher Power. Thus, we can assume it's God's will for us to keep attending meetings regularly, even when we don't feel like it. Or, when we're in a group of people who are gossiping about someone we dislike, we might be inclined to join in with a few comments of our own at first. But we've learned from experience that gossip is not good for us, so we know it's God's will that we not take part in the damaging conversation. Honesty, common sense, and a sincere willingness to follow our new spiritual path are sufficient to show us the way.

In making major decisions, of course, we should not assume that every thought that comes into our minds is inspired by God. When we're considering taking an unusual action, we will want to consult with a sponsor or spiritual guide. It is not this person's job to decide for us; no human can do that. But a person who is detached from our immediate situation and has an understanding of spiritual principles can help us to learn and apply them when we are searching for our Higher Power's will for us.

This, then, is how we will operate our lives, once we have made the decision called for in Step Three. None of us can follow this way of life perfectly, but we find that our success in recovery and our freedom from food obsession are in direct proportion to how sincerely we try to live in this manner.

Taking Step Three shows our willingness to live by God's will, one day at a time. Most of us have found that working the Twelve Steps and applying them in our lives has helped us better understand God's will. Having this willingness to work the Steps, we do not let any doubt or confusion we may still have keep us from acting. We concentrate on whomever or whatever we think God might be, and we say out loud, in words of our own choosing, that we now turn our will and our lives over to our Higher Power, holding nothing back.

When we say our personal prayer asking for help, and mean it, we have made the key, life-changing decision that will lead us to recovery. We have taken the Third Step. We now have a new reaction when we face a problem or a decision, whether it has to do with food, life, or our own runaway emotions. Instead of acting on impulse, we pause long enough to learn God's will. Then, instead of resorting to willpower, we relax and reach out to receive help from our Higher Power. All we need to say is, "God, please help me do your will."

Once we compulsive eaters truly take the Third Step, we cannot fail to recover. As we live out our decision day by day, our Higher Power guides us through the remaining nine Steps. When we falter, we are reminded of our commitment to live by God's will alone, and we trust that the willingness and ability will come if we only ask for them. When we get off track, our Higher Power will guide us back, as long as we are sincerely trying to know and do God's will. We can confidently face any situation life brings because we no longer have to face it alone. We have what we need any time we are willing to let go of self-will and humbly ask for help.

# STEP FOUR

Made a searching and fearless moral inventory
of ourselves.

---

*SPIRITUAL PRINCIPLE*

## COURAGE

In Step Four we take an honest look at the beliefs, attitudes, values, and behaviors that lead us to the food. How we choose to look at and deal with our lives and the world lies at the core of the disease. We need to consider such things as self-centeredness, anger, resentment, fear, pride, dishonesty, and negative thinking as well as our sexual attitudes and behaviors.

Those of us who have completed Step Four have found that taking this searching and fearless moral inventory was one of the most loving things we have ever done for ourselves. As we took an honest look at the past, we began to understand ourselves better. That understanding was the beginning of emotional healing. Many of us had lived our lives up to this point with a secret feeling of shame. We carried deep in our hearts the feeling that we were worthless or insignificant. Often, this shame stemmed from unresolved guilt over mistakes we'd never fully dealt with. We had never faced our wrongs honestly and acknowledged them, so we were left with feelings of shame or guilt. Writing our Step Four inventory has enabled us to begin cleaning up the messes of the past so we can start life over, afresh.

The self-analysis we do in Step Four is essential to our recovery from compulsive eating. This Step continues the transformation process that began with our admission of powerlessness in Step One, a process of increasing honesty and self-awareness that will gradually free us from our bondage to self. Our past problems have been controlling our actions and feelings for years, often in ways of which we are not aware. As we face the problems, they lose their power to overwhelm and control us. We no longer have the need to protect ourselves from uncomfortable feelings by eating compulsively or using other destructive food behaviors.

We have found it best to approach this inventory with the words "fearless" and "searching" uppermost in our minds. Many of us have become experts in self-deception after years of lying to ourselves about how much we have been eating and the problems our eating behaviors have caused us physically, emotionally, and spiritually. We've lied to ourselves about our other problems, too, denying that we've made mistakes, that we've been wrong about things, that we need to change. We *must* change if we are to recover. Change begins with honesty. As we work the Fourth Step, we develop a new ability to see our own dishonesty and a greater willingness to live by truth.

Ideally, we take our Step Four inventory after we have stopped eating compulsively, so that we have the clarity of mind to be thorough in our self-examination. By having a plan of eating, working with a sponsor, and using all of OA's other Tools, we are better able to become and stay abstinent, one day at a time, while doing our Fourth Step.

Delaying the Fourth Step until we feel we can do it "perfectly" only delays our recovery. Some of us spent months seeking advice from sponsors, friends, and people at meetings, studying all sorts of literature on the subject, looking for the one "right" way to do Step Four. When our sponsors told us, "the important thing is just to *do* it," we didn't understand. Until we took the Fourth Step, we didn't realize that perfectionism was one of our troublesome defects of character.

Some of us delayed beginning Step Four simply because we didn't want to do it. We realize being *willing* to do the inventory and *wanting* to do it are two different things. The Twelve Steps are a process for change. This inventory and the rest of the Steps are the implementation of our Step Three commitment. The decision we made to "turn our will and our lives over" to a Power greater than ourselves is meaningless unless it is followed by action.

Sometimes we began the program with enthusiasm but fell back into the disease while waiting for the desire to do Step Four to overtake us. We have found that a simple prayer for willingness to take action works to get us started on our inventory.

We then make a commitment to ourselves, our Higher Power, and our sponsors to work on the inventory regularly until it is completed. We might also want to review the questions in *The Twelve-Step Workbook of Overeaters Anonymous,* which are designed to help us get started. Any action, no matter how small, can help us overcome procrastination.

We have found it is necessary to write our inventory. Anyone who has taken an inventory in a store or other business can verify that it is difficult to keep track of what is in stock unless it is written down. The writing process helps us to examine the feelings that are connected to our actions. We begin to see clearly how some of our reactions had served us well while others had unbalanced us emotionally, setting up patterns of negative thinking and self-destructive behavior.

Sometimes we began a Step Four inventory without knowing why it was necessary, doing it simply because we had been told it would help us recover from compulsive eating. We tried it and it worked. This is one example of what we mean when we say that in OA we learn to utilize, not analyze.

Those of us who tried to analyze the Step soon found we were wasting time. Nor did it help to analyze ourselves before we did the Step. It worked far better when we plunged in and started writing.

What form should our inventory take? Any form at all. There is no one right way, since we are writing for ourselves and are never required to show our inventory to anyone. In fact, we find that *how* we do the Fourth Step inventory makes little difference. What counts most is that we do it. When we write it, we need to focus on our thinking and behaviors, past and present, that have caused us difficulties. Our sponsors can help by suggesting ways to approach our inventory, and can serve as an invaluable sounding board during the writing process.

One way is to use the guidelines set forth in the Big Book.[2] For a complete explanation of that method, refer to *Alcoholics Anonymous, Fourth Edition,* pages 64–71.

Another way is to use the *Twelve Step Workshop and Study Guide* of Overeaters Anonymous.

A third way is to conduct our inventory by asking ourselves questions about specific character traits and behaviors, such as self-centeredness, anger, resentment, fear, pride, dishonesty, negative thinking, shame, guilt, and sexual attitudes and behaviors. Then we examine in writing the ways that we've exhibited these characteristics in our lives.

## Self-Centeredness

*In what ways have I been power hungry?*

*In what ways have I tried to control my spouse, partner, parents, brothers or sisters, children, friends, employers, colleagues, teachers, or others?*

*How have I manipulated people?*

*In what ways have I intimidated others?*

*How has jealousy caused me to be possessive of a mate or friend?*

---

[2] *Alcoholics Anonymous,* 4th ed. (Alcoholics Anonymous World Services, Inc., © 2001).

*How have I reacted when I don't get my way or when people disagree with me?*

*In what ways have I been defiant, either openly or secretly? What has been my attitude toward laws, rules, and people who have legitimate authority over me?*

*In what ways have I been intolerant of differences?*

*How have I created or perpetuated conflict with others?*

*In what ways have I insisted on being the center of attention? How have I acted offensively just to be noticed?*

*When have I acted selfishly, letting my own desires govern me while I ignore the needs of others?*

*When have I spent money my family needed in order to feed my illness or gratify my desires?*

*At what times or under what circumstances have I been unavailable to my children or my mate when they needed me?*

*How has greed affected my life? In what ways have I been selfish or dissatisfied with what I have, always wanting more?*

*Have I been obsessed with money? If so, what behaviors have I exhibited? In what ways have I thought money will solve my problems?*

*In what ways have I been lazy and slothful?*

*Have I done my share in the work of groups of which I'm a member? If not, why not?*

*When have I been oversensitive, quick to take offense at what people say to me? When have I laughed everything off, pretending nothing hurts me?*

*In what ways have I procrastinated or attempted to be perfect? What actions have I delayed because of my perfectionism?*

*When have I abandoned someone I had a responsibility to help?*

*How often have I taken on other people's responsibilities, doing for them the things they should be doing for themselves?*

*In what ways have I been willing to take responsibility for the problems I cause? When have I tried to shift the blame to others?*

*When have I rationalized my misbehavior?*

*Have I been overly dependent on others? In what ways have I tried to avoid responsibility for my actions? In what ways have I depended on others to take care of me?*

## Anger/Resentment

*In what circumstances have I avoided dealing with anger and resentment by resorting to compulsive food behaviors?*

*In what ways have I held onto grudges because someone threatened or damaged my self-esteem, security, ambitions, or relationships? How have I tried to get even with people who hurt me? What has been the effect of never forgetting when someone harms me?*

*When have I held a grudge against someone due to jealousy? In what ways have I been envious of other people's appearance, wealth, sex life, popularity, possessions, or position in society?*

*In what ways have I resented myself for things I did or failed to do, or for being a compulsive eater?*

*How have I tended to be harsh, unforgiving, and self-righteous?*

*How have I misdirected my anger or lashed out at those closest to me? Why have I been unable to tell someone that I am angry or annoyed at him or her?*

*In what ways have I abused another person verbally, emotionally, or physically?*

*Have I mistreated any animals, and if so, in what way?*

*Have I ever taken anyone's life because of my anger, fear, carelessness, or other reason? What happened?*

### Fear

*In what ways have I been anxious about the future? How much of my time have I spent worrying?*

*In what ways have I been afraid of people? How have I isolated myself from friends or society?*

*Have I been afraid to reach out to others? How have I held back, waiting for them to come to me?*

*In what ways have I gotten into relationships with people who abuse me?*

*In what circumstances have I been afraid to end existing relationships that are destructive or inappropriate for me?*

*How have worry and fear kept me from seeking a new job or career? In what ways have I been so afraid of change that I remain in situations that are not good for me?*

*How have fear, worry, and anxiety affected my life? What people, places, and institutions have I feared? How has fear driven me to compulsive food behaviors?*

*Have I been afraid to express myself, to tell others how I feel? How has that affected me?*

*Have I been so afraid of conflict that I accept abuse rather than risk asserting myself? In what ways has this affected me?*

*When has fear held me back from taking actions I might have pursued?*

*When have I stood by and allowed another person to be hurt when I could have done something to prevent it? In what ways have I let another person be blamed or punished for something I did?*

*Have I trusted people, or have I had faith in no one, including myself? How have others let me down? How have I let myself down?*

*Have I been bigoted? Have I ever denied anyone fair treatment because of race, religion, politics, gender, sexual orientation, or disability? Have I told ethnic, racist, or sexist jokes? If not, have I* been afraid to say that I don't enjoy such "humor"? How has this kept me from accepting others?

## Pride/False Pride

*How have arrogance and false pride characterized my behavior? How has pride caused me to act?*

*Have I been a people-pleaser? Have I needed everybody to like me, so much so that I make it my goal to find out what people want and give it to them, no matter the cost to myself? Have I been afraid to say no to others? In what ways has this harmed me or others?*

*In what ways have I indulged in self-pity? When have I played the martyr?*

*Have I let the needs of others govern me while I ignore my own needs? How has this harmed me?*

*In what ways have I been afraid of not being recognized, respected, or loved? Why have I been afraid that I won't get my share or that people won't listen to me? How have I insisted on being first? How has prideful self-centeredness caused me to act?*

*Have I been a status-seeker? How much money, time, and energy have I spent trying to impress or show myself to be better than others?*

*In what ways have I been a snob? Have I treated some people better than others based on their status?*

*What actions have I taken to put people down or put them in their place?*

*Have I had a tendency to belittle others? Why have I done this?*

*Have I ever played a mean trick on someone? What were the consequences of my actions?*

*In what ways have I condemned people for things I also have done? When have I been a hypocrite, even while denouncing the hypocrisy of others?*

*How have I tried to harm another's reputation?*

*Have I indulged in gossip or listened to and enjoyed the gossip of others? Why have I done this and how has it been harmful to myself and others?*

*Have I admitted my mistakes and acknowledged that others are sometimes right? Have I been teachable or complacent?*

## Dishonesty

*In what ways have I been dishonest and unworthy of trust?*

*When have I been sneaky or practiced deception? How have I taken advantage of someone's ignorance instead of telling the full truth?*

*When have I kept money or items I found instead of returning them to their rightful owners?*

*When have I taken money, food, or other things that didn't belong to me?*

*Have I ever damaged anyone's property and not repaired or paid for the damage?*

*In what situations have I borrowed things and not returned them?*

*When have I broken a confidence? Why and what were the consequences?*

*When have I cheated on tests or in games or contests?*

*When and how have I cheated others?*

*When and how have I cheated and lied to myself?*

*In what ways have I lived in denial about my eating, character defects, or need to change?*

## Negative Thinking

*Have I tended to dwell on dark thoughts? How has that affected my life and the lives of others?*

*Have I been thankful for what I have, or have I ignored my blessings and focused on what I lack? If so, how has that affected my life?*

*Have I been optimistic or pessimistic? Have I concentrated on the positive, or have I become obsessed with bad things that might happen? How has this affected me?*

*How has my negative outlook made life bleak for others who live and work with me? When have I been cynical and critical?*

*Have I accepted my own failings and those of others as natural, or have I criticized, condemned, and complained? What have been the consequences?*

## Shame

*Where has shame been a factor in my life?*

*How have I felt about having the disease of compulsive eating and my issues around willpower?*

*How have I felt about my body and intimacy?*

*In what ways have I berated myself and my achievements?*

*In what ways have I compared myself to others?*

## Guilt

*What have I considered the worst things I've done in my life? Why do I still feel guilty about these things?*

*In what ways have I not forgiven myself and moved on?*

*What secrets have I kept that I need to share so I can move forward, free and unencumbered?*

## Sexual Attitudes and Behaviors

*What problems has sex caused me?*

*In what ways have I pursued sex that damaged my self-esteem? When have I been promiscuous?*

*When have my sexual fantasies interfered with my ability to build relationships? In what ways have I chosen fantasy, shutting out my partner or spouse?*

*How have I been interested only in my own pleasure, never seeking to please my sexual partner as well?*

*How have I sought to satisfy my sexual impulses at the expense of others?*

*When have I had an inappropriate intimate relationship with another person's spouse or partner? When have I cheated on my own spouse or partner?*

*How have I forced or manipulated someone to have sexual contact with me?*

*Have I ever sexually molested anyone? Have I ever had sexual contact with a child or anyone who was not fully capable of consenting? Explain.*

*In what instances have I abused a position of trust to get sex from someone who sought my help?*

*In what ways have I used intimidation or abused a position of power to get sex? When have I threatened or sought revenge against someone who wouldn't go along with my sexual advances?*

*Have I used sex or pregnancy to manipulate or trap someone in a relationship? What were my motives? What were the results of my actions?*

*Have I ever gotten someone pregnant and not shared responsibility for the outcome? What were the consequences?*

*Have I transmitted a disease when I knew I was infected? What can I do about this now?*

*In what other ways have I misused my sexual drives?*

*In what ways has compulsive eating made me uninterested in sex? In what ways have I been unfair to my partner(s) and myself, preferring isolation and food to the risk of physical intimacy?*

We have answered many questions and identified many short-comings to be addressed in later Steps. But no matter how many shortcomings we have, it's important to recognize that we have many good qualities as well. Now is the time to make a list of our positive characteristics.

As we look at our assets, we may want to remember that no one is perfect. For example, am I generally accepting, agreeable, authentic, charitable, compassionate, considerate, and courteous? Am I ethical, faithful, forgiving, grateful, generous, helpful, honor-able, and hopeful? Some other assets to consider are industrious, kind, loving, loyal, patient, positive, productive, respectful, sincere, thoughtful, tolerant, and understanding.

After writing our inventory, we review it. Have we listed every-thing we can think of about ourselves, destructive as well as con-structive? We've found that we need to write down all of our charac-teristics, tendencies, feelings, prejudices, and actions we have taken as a result. Some of our actions are painful for us to recall, but we write them down anyway. When we face the guilt that truthfully tells us, "You made a mistake," we're freed of shame that falsely tells us, "You *are* a mistake."

Once we've made the inventory, checked it, and reviewed it, we ask God to help us remember anything more that belongs there. We spend some time in quiet meditation, concentrating on our com-plete willingness to face whatever truths about ourselves God wants to show us. If we realize we have left out an important item, we add it to our inventory. As we continue toward recovery, we'll find more shortcomings and more positive characteristics. Right now, how-ever, all we need to do is list everything we are aware of at present.

Looking over what we have written, we shouldn't be discour-aged if the negative outweighs the positive. After all, if we found nothing wrong, we wouldn't need our program of recovery. In fact, we've found that the more defects we uncover, the more our lives can improve as we continue working the Twelve Steps.

Each of us who completes a Fourth Step inventory in OA finds it essential to our recovery and a major factor in changing our lives.

As we reach the end of Step Four, we discover that a promise made in Our Invitation to You[3] has begun to be fulfilled. We are "moving beyond the food and the emotional havoc to a fuller living experience."[4]

---

[3] *Overeaters Anonymous,* 3rd ed. (Overeaters Anonymous, Inc., © 1980 ... 2014) pp. 1-5.
[4] Ibid. p. 2.

# STEP FIVE

Admitted to God, to ourselves,
and to another human being the exact nature
of our wrongs.

---

*SPIRITUAL PRINCIPLE*

**INTEGRITY**

Throughout our lives, many of us have felt isolated from other people. We felt that we were outsiders, and we acted out this feeling in many ways, some of us by being shy, others by being arrogant or belligerent, others by playing the clown. No matter how we acted, however, deep down we felt alone and apart. Now, looking at the Fifth Step, we see something we can do—a positive action that we can take—to end our isolation.

By the time we reach this point in our OA program, most of us are already feeling less alone. Since joining Overeaters Anonymous, we've learned to accept the loving welcome we've found in our meetings and are now part of the Fellowship. We've talked with others over the phone, reached out through digital communication, shared at meetings, and discussed our lives in depth with our sponsors. We've begun to make true friends in OA, friends with whom we can speak honestly. Perhaps it has become easier to share about how we acted while we were eating compulsively. On a deeper level, however, we probably realize that there is still much of ourselves we haven't shared. This is natural.

Few of us had ever done a moral inventory before we joined OA, and our Fourth Step inventory brought us new insights and understandings. By the time we have completed the Fourth Step, most of us feel ready to move ahead quickly with Step Five. We want to be free of the resentments, guilt, and shame rooted in the past, and we realize that sharing the details of our past with another human being is an important step toward freedom. Once we have taken this Step, we will no longer have anything to hide. This is the beginning of the end of our isolation.

Step Five starts with our Higher Power. Most of us find that without the help of a Power greater than ourselves we are incapable of accepting that it was our attitudes and actions that led to so many of our problems. It is human nature to cling to the illusion that we have done no wrong, and through the years, we have become experts at rationalizing our thoughts and behaviors. Now, with God's help, we leave rationalization behind and begin to practice integrity. We face the reality of what we've done. We see the part we have played in creating our own misfortunes and realize the futility of continuing to blame others for our eating behaviors and unmanageable lives.

In Step Five we continue to learn there can be a new way to live. From now on, we readily acknowledge our shortcomings instead of seeking to hide them from ourselves and others. A humble admission of our mistakes to God is our first step in this new direction. We willingly open our hearts so that a life-changing Power can come in and heal us. We go back over our Fourth Step inventory, acknowledging each truth about our past behaviors, no matter how painful or embarrassing. In acknowledging to God these truths about our past, we begin at last to acknowledge them to ourselves, too. We admit to ourselves who we've been and what we've done. As we do this, we gain new hope. We start to feel that we can forgive ourselves, be forgiven, and move toward creating a new life, free from food obsession.

Once we have made the admissions to God and to ourselves, we may feel we have fully dealt with our past. What need is there, we may ask, to share our deep, hidden secrets with another person? Won't this self-revelation simply humiliate us and further lower our already low self-esteem?

In practice, when we actually share our Fifth Step, we find that we are humbled without being humiliated. Many of us have felt that we had to be better than everybody else or we were no good at all. Through the Fifth Step process, we begin to see reality. All our striving to get ahead has been useless. We are neither above nor below the rest of the human race; we are a part of it, shaped by the same basic needs and desires as all our fellows. Those of us who have belittled ourselves or felt we were worse than others also gain a new perspective. In sharing honestly with another person, we begin to feel a sense of relief. Someone knows all about us and still accepts us unconditionally. We begin to forgive ourselves and see ourselves as capable, strong, and honest. And so we are: In taking Step Five, we prove ourselves capable of accomplishing a difficult task and strong enough to be completely honest.

Admitting the exact nature of our wrongs to another person can be a frightening prospect, for we've never before risked such complete openness. Yet, we find that we haven't really admitted the full truth to ourselves until we speak about it with someone else. It is only through the process of discussing our shortcomings with an understanding person that we can finally begin to know and accept ourselves. Nothing in us can be changed until we first accept it. Step Five, by helping us to know and accept ourselves, makes it possible for us to change and recover.

It is important to choose a trustworthy and understanding person with whom to complete Step Five. For many of us that person is the sponsor who helped us take the first four Steps of the program. Some of us have found that we feel more comfortable confiding in a person other than our sponsor. Either is acceptable, so long as it is right for us. We understand that if we pick a person other than our sponsor, we are not rejecting our sponsor.

Any person who is recovering in a Twelve Step fellowship and who has completed the Fifth Step is usually a good choice to listen to our Fifth Step. Such a person can easily understand what we are trying to accomplish with Step Five. However, there is no rule that says we cannot share our Fifth Step with someone outside the program—a therapist, for instance, or a religious counselor. We ask for God's guidance, give the matter some thought, and then move ahead with action.

We are not looking for someone to tell us how to solve our problems. What we need is a loving witness, someone who can keep our confidences and listen without judging us or seeking to fix us. Also, we want to confide in someone who can be objective enough to tell us if there's something glaring we've omitted and can guide us through this process if needed. Step Five is usually our first attempt to fully open our hearts to another human being. Most of us need loving guidance in learning this new skill.

When working this Step, we do more than just recite thoughts, words, and actions from the past that we consider to be our wrongs. We need to discuss the "exact nature" of those wrongs. This means we need to talk about the feelings, thoughts and beliefs that led to our actions as well as how we felt afterward. We need to look at what those actions have cost us. For instance, it's not enough to acknowledge that we have held a grudge against a certain person; we also need to talk about what it is in our nature that has caused us to react that way. Have we been jealous? Have we been resentful because of our thwarted desire to control another person? Then we discuss how these negative feelings and actions have affected us materially, emotionally, and spiritually.

Sometimes, coming to understand our motives helps us to forgive ourselves. Often we see that, at some level, we were fighting for survival when we did the things we did. Most of us find that fear is at the root of many of our damaging emotions and actions. As we grow in the Twelve Step way of life, we learn that our fears usually stem from our inability to trust that our basic needs will be met. Perhaps we have good reasons for our mistrust; perhaps people have failed us, placing us in situations we were not emotionally prepared to handle. Still, we find we have to outgrow our doubts. If we are to recover, we must learn to trust other people and entrust our lives to a Power greater than ourselves.

Learning this kind of trust is a gradual process. Our Fifth Step is a giant stride forward. By opening our past and sharing our deepest secrets, we are making ourselves vulnerable in a way we have not been since childhood.

Can we trust that this person won't use this knowledge to hurt us? Determined to get well, we willingly take the risk. When we do, a miracle happens. Another individual knows us truly and fully, yet accepts us anyway. We begin to experience trust, and we feel that if another person can accept us unconditionally perhaps we can accept ourselves unconditionally as well.

Sometimes, during the process of doing Steps Four and Five, we become aware of more than our character defects. Sometimes we uncover old traumas: Experiences of being abandoned, abused, sexually molested, or raped are far more common among us than anybody would like to believe. These and other memories have been so deeply painful to those of us who were victims that we have spent our lives running from them and eating to cover them up. Until we began to deal with them, some of us found that our abstinence was precarious or we continued to feel unhappy, even while we were abstaining and working the Steps. In such cases, some of us have looked for help from qualified professionals and groups, in addition to working the program. Many have found that therapy alone doesn't permanently solve our eating problems. We need to continue with the Twelve Steps and OA for lasting abstinence and recovery.

You may find it useful at the end of your Fifth Step to make a list of your key shortcomings, perhaps with the help of the person taking your Fifth Step. This will help to prepare you for Steps Six and Seven.

As we complete Step Five, we may feel many emotions, among them humility, elation, and relief. We often feel nearer than ever before to our Higher Power and more loving and trusting of other people. Whether we feel these things or not, we can rest assured that we *are* nearer to God and more capable of trusting others. The fruits of having faithfully completed Step Five may be apparent immediately or gradually, but they will appear. Taking Step Five is the beginning of freedom, and as we continue working the Steps, the great burden of our past actions will be lifted from us. We find we can face each day and each challenge as it comes.

In the process of sharing our inventory, we have become more honest with ourselves and others than we have ever been before. Honesty is a key factor in our recovery from compulsive eating, and so we will want to develop this trait. The best way to do so is to continue working the Twelve Steps. In this way, we can learn how to deal with those troubling aspects of ourselves that we discovered in Steps Four and Five. Simply knowing what is wrong with us isn't always enough. Steps Six through Twelve show us more actions we can take to bring about the necessary changes in our lives. From this point on, we begin to leave behind the character defects that have caused us so many problems in the past.

# STEP SIX

Were entirely ready to have God remove all these
defects of character.

---

*SPIRITUAL PRINCIPLE*

## WILLINGNESS

At first glance, Step Six seems easy. After all, who among us
would not want to have all our defects miraculously removed, once we have identified them? As soon as possible, we want
to get on with the business of being perfect people. Many of us are
tempted to pass quickly over this Step without giving it due thought.

"Go ahead, God!" we say. "I'm entirely ready." Then we swear off
the old self-destructive behaviors, only to find ourselves right back
in their grip within a short time. "I *know* better than this!" we berate
ourselves. Our character defects seem to stick to us like glue as we
try time and again to turn them over to God.

In practice, Step Six may be one of the most difficult of the
Twelve Steps, because we find that *saying* we're entirely ready and
*being* entirely ready to take action are two very different things.

What we are entirely ready for, actually, is to have the difficulties our defects have caused us removed while we hang on to the defects themselves.

Why is it so hard for us to be entirely ready to part with our defects? For many of us, the reason is fear. We are comfortable with our old ways of thinking and acting, even though we know they are harmful. We have no idea what life would look like or how we would handle feelings without them because we've never known how to cope with life any other way. Often we feel we'd be less interesting as human beings without some of our defects. While we don't enjoy the pain they have often caused us, they are so much a part of us that the thought of having them suddenly removed is threatening to us. Perhaps resentments have dominated our thinking for so long that we don't know what else to think about. Or, maybe we're afraid that if God eliminates our cynicism, lying, and gossiping, we'll be left with nothing interesting to talk about. We admit that our old ways of relating to other people have caused pain and we want to let go of them. But how *will* we act? In honestly facing Step Six, we confront the fear that our defects are like threads woven into the very fabric of our being; if God removes them, we feel we'll surely unravel.

Often we face an even more difficult obstacle. Some of our destructive thinking and behaviors are not only familiar and comfortable to us, they're also enjoyable. We get a rush of excitement from telling a lie and getting away with it, so we say to ourselves our falsehoods, after all, are harmless "white" lies. Our fantasies make us feel important, so we overlook how they waste the time we could be using to deal with our real lives. We enjoy picking up juicy tidbits of gossip and passing them on, so we rationalize that the people we're talking about deserve it, they'll never find out, or everyone does it. Some of us get a charge out of having a fight or throwing a temper tantrum and the control over other people that these outbursts have usually gained us. Say what we will about being "completely ready" in a general way to have God remove our shortcomings, when it comes to specifics, we'd rather hang on to a few of our favorites.

For these reasons, we're tempted to rationalize the defect itself.

"After all, nobody expects us to be perfect," we say. "We strive for progress, not perfection." Such reasoning only delays our recovery. The Sixth Step calls for us to be *entirely* ready to have God remove *all* our defects of character. Those of us who take this Step with the total commitment required to make it work do indeed strive for the ultimate refinement of our character.

Even when we do approach Step Six with complete willingness, another problem often arises. Some of us misunderstand this Step and act as if we can remove our shortcomings on our own, rather than asking God for help. In our attempts to be rid of dishonesty, for instance, we may try to reform and become brutally honest. Or, we see we've been selfish, so we try to be overly generous. If anger is one of our problems, we try never to get angry. Or, if we've heard that fear is incompatible with faith, we try not to feel any fear.

All these are good efforts, but they often seem to get us nowhere. The harder we try to rid ourselves of our defects, the more they control us. Because we have misread Step Six, we feel totally defeated in our attempts to work it. Thus we learn a key truth about ourselves and our Twelve Step program. We are powerless over each of our defects of character, just as we are powerless over the food. Our character defects need to be removed by a Power greater than ourselves; we cannot do it alone.

Does this mean we shouldn't try to change our behavior until our Higher Power changes us? Should we continue being dishonest, intolerant, and all the rest? Of course not. Being "entirely ready" means that we firmly turn our backs on the old self-destructive behaviors and make every effort to live by the Principles embodied in the Twelve Steps. Trying to practice the new thinking and behaviors to the best of our ability shows our true willingness to change.

But neither should we become discouraged if we find that we aren't changing as quickly as we would like. We can't expect to be free of all our defects overnight. What we are asked to do in Step Six is to become entirely ready for this miracle of release to happen to us, no matter what it may cost us, no matter what in our lives may change.

When we work Step Six, we dedicate ourselves to a lifetime of growth and change. Being entirely ready means we are completely willing to recognize and let go of our defective behavior patterns, and to let God change us as God will. We don't set the timetable or method for these changes. When and how our defects are removed is entirely up to God. Our work is to do what we can to make ourselves ready, by actively reaching for recovery and putting ourselves in the frame of mind to receive God's help.

We might begin to do this by submitting each defect to close scrutiny. In Steps Four and Five, we took a long hard look at each trait and acknowledged it as a part of our lives. Now we ask ourselves what it is doing *for* us as well as what it is doing *to* us. We search out our reasons for hanging on to each trait. Perhaps one has been a readily available source of comfort, while another has added excitement to our lives, and a third has enabled us to compensate for our lack of self-esteem. Every character defect we have today has been useful to us at some point in our lives, and we need to recognize that fact.

Next, we need to recognize that each of these old tools for coping with life has now outlived its usefulness. We look at the harm we are doing to ourselves by clinging to each of these ways of thinking and acting. We had to "hit bottom" in order to look at our eating behavior and, now we have to do the same with each of these traits. Only when we fully realize that the defects of character are costing us more than they are giving us will we become entirely ready to be rid of our destructive thinking and behaviors.

Working the Sixth Step is a lot like working the first Three Steps on each of our defects. We remind ourselves: "I'm powerless to rid myself of this trait. I can't, but God can. I'll let God take it."

A willingness to change is the essence of Step Six. Change is always frightening, even when it's a much-needed and long-overdue change for the better. Many of us have wasted years and suffered a lot of pain in order to avoid having to change. As we work Step Six, we recognize and acknowledge our human fear of change. Then, because we are willing to go to any length for recovery from compulsive eating, we move ahead with this Step anyhow. No longer will we allow fear to keep us from doing what is best for us. After all, we have confronted the first Five Steps, taken them in spite of our fear, and lived to tell the story. By the time we reach Step Six, we're almost used to doing the very things we've been the most afraid of.

As with the five earlier Steps, our rewards when we've taken Step Six are great. Although we may not realize it at first, our commitment to embrace the needed changes in our thinking and behavior has given us an extraordinary power to deal with life's challenges. No longer do we go through each day clinging desperately to the past, resistant to change. From now on, we strive to keep ourselves entirely ready for any transformations our Higher Power wants to bring about in us. Having such an attitude, we cannot fail. We become wiser, saner, more effective people as we recover from the disease of compulsive eating. We find we can cope with both good times and bad, learning and growing spiritually from each experience, as our Higher Power intended us to do all along.

# STEP SEVEN

Humbly asked Him to remove our shortcomings.

---

*SPIRITUAL PRINCIPLE*

## HUMILITY

Having become completely ready to let go of our character defects in Step Six, we find that Step Seven is simple; all we have to do is ask God to remove our shortcomings. There is a qualification, however. As we ask, Step Seven calls for us to adopt an attitude of humility.

Many of us misunderstood the concept of humility at first; we confused it with humiliation or low self-esteem. We felt we had suffered enough humiliation to last a lifetime, and we balked when our sponsors or fellow members suggested we might need to become more humble. We felt that humility was not what we needed, since low self-esteem had been a large part of our problem. In OA we learned that low self-esteem was not at all the same as humility. In fact, a poor self-image keeps us in bondage to self and thus makes it impossible for us to find true humility.

As we began to recover in OA, we could see how compulsive eating had caused us to be obsessed with ourselves and our status. Humiliated by our inability to control our intake of food and by the devastating consequences of compulsive eating behaviors, we fought for self-esteem with all our might. As our disease progressed and our compulsive eating worsened, our self-esteem fell progressively lower, and we fought ever harder to bolster it by gaining whatever mastery we could over our fellow beings. In our self-absorption, we became status seekers in one way or another. Primarily concerned with getting our own way and the recognition we craved, we tried openly or secretly to place ourselves above other people, hoping to disprove our own feelings of inadequacy.

In OA, we have discovered that humility is simply an awareness of who we really are today and a willingness to become all that we can be. Genuine humility brings an end to the feelings of inadequacy, the self-absorption, and the status seeking. Humility, as we encounter it in our OA Fellowship, places us neither above nor below other people on some imagined ladder of worth. It places us exactly where we belong, on an equal footing with our fellow beings and in harmony with God.

If we have earnestly worked the first six Steps of the program, we have already come a long way toward this new attitude of humility. We have admitted our need for help as we have begun to let go of self-will, have become willing to acknowledge our true selves—defects and all—and have become willing to have our self-defeating attitudes and traits changed. Before we ask our Higher Power for these changes with genuine humility, there are several concepts we need to understand.

First, we are not asking God to remove our shortcomings so that we can be better than other people. That kind of self-righteousness would be a step backward in our journey of recovery. Self-righteousness motivates us when we find ourselves looking down on others who are not working the Twelve Steps, whether they are people outside OA or members of our Fellowship. As we take Step Seven, our goal is simply to draw closer to being the people God intends us to be. We pray to be made new, not for our own gratification, but so that we may be more useful instruments of our Higher Power.

Second, often a shortcoming isn't removed immediately, or it returns after being gone for a while. Every one of us has experienced struggles with some of our character defects, even after praying for their removal. The existence of the struggle is not a sign that we lack humility. But what attitude do we take during these difficult times? If we are surprised, shocked, deflated, or discouraged when a defect returns, we lack humility. If we get angry at God, ourselves, or other people because we have the defect, we lack humility. Real humility about our character defects carries with it *acceptance*. We accept that each defect, as painful to us as it may be, is a part of who we are. With humble acceptance we can quietly say to our Higher Power, "I am this way, and only with your help can I change."

However, humility means that we aren't smug when a defect that has long been a part of our lives is removed; we're genuinely relieved. We recognize our release from the defect as a miracle, evidence of the power of God's healing love, and we are honestly grateful. Instead of approaching those who still suffer a similar problem with an attitude of superiority, we offer them hope. They may well say to themselves, "If she (or he) can change, surely I can too!"

Obviously, this kind of humility is not something we can learn simply by willing ourselves to be humble.

Humility is a gift as surely as is our recovery from compulsive eating and the other miracles of healing we experience as we work the Twelve Steps. Our job is to be willing to let go of old attitudes that block humility, such as low self-esteem, status seeking, and self-righteousness.

Our approach to Step Seven, then, might begin with a prayer for genuine humility. Having said this prayer, we can proceed with the rest of Step Seven, trusting that our Higher Power will grant us the gift of humility to a greater and greater degree as we continue to let go of our old values and practice the Principles of the Twelve Steps, one day at a time. We don't have to wait until we achieve perfect humility to proceed with Step Seven and the remaining five Steps.

We proceed with our Step Seven prayer, secure in the knowledge that we are doing our part and God will do the rest.

How do we work Step Seven? Quite simply, we take our written inventory or list of character defects in hand. (Some of us have found it helpful to assume a physical posture of humility as we pray.) With our list before us, we name each shortcoming individually and ask God to deal with it whenever and however God wants. We express our complete willingness to have each shortcoming removed from us. We express our desire to become more effective in serving and helping others as our shortcomings are transformed into assets. Having done this, we have taken Step Seven.[5]

Can we now expect to miraculously become perfect beings? Probably not. In fact, as we continue with the Twelve Steps, we will almost certainly discover defects we didn't see during the house-cleaning we undertook in Steps Four through Seven. Humility means we will no longer be shocked and horrified when we realize we have yet another defect. We begin with the premise that there could be many things about us that need to change, only some of which we're able to see at any given time. In God's time, when God knows we're ready, we will be given new insights into our true defects of character—we will, that is, if we are honestly working our program. When this happens, we apply the Principles of the program, including those of Steps Six and Seven, willingness and humility. We fully acknowledge and accept the shortcoming as belonging to us. We then examine our motives and the effect this behavior is having on our lives until we are sure we're ready to let go of it. We acknowledge our powerlessness to remove the defect ourselves and humbly ask God to take it from us; then we get up and go on with life in a new frame of mind, knowing that God will indeed remove the shortcoming.

Often we are shown actions that we are to take as each defect is being removed. For instance, we may visualize ourselves as the people we will be when we no longer have each particular defect.

---

[5] The Big Book Step Seven Prayer is found in *Alcoholics Anonymous,* 4th ed. (Alcoholics Anonymous World Services, Inc., © 2001) p. 76.

How will we think and act? We may find it helpful to rehearse what we'll say and do when tempted to act in the old self-destructive ways. Sometimes we may be caught off guard and fall back into the defective patterns, but if we persist in visualizing and practicing better ways of life, they will, with our Higher Power's help, eventually become second nature. When we make a mistake, we acknowledge that fact without claiming that we ourselves *are* that mistake. From now on, we cease telling ourselves we are always going to be dishonest, selfish, abusive, stupid, or bad people. Instead, we repeatedly affirm the truth about ourselves—that we are becoming honest, caring, nurturing, wise, and effective human beings as we practice our new behaviors, day by day.

These actions may seem like hard work at first, but we've found that our willingness to act is an important factor in our healing. It indicates our sincerity. Are we willing to make an investment of time and energy to change our attitudes and actions? To what lengths are we willing to go in order to be rid of these shortcomings? Effort on our part will help us to appreciate the miracle we are about to receive, rather than to take it for granted. Yet when the miracle happens, we know for certain that we didn't simply get better by ourselves. We have taken action under the guidance of our Higher Power, and God has worked through us to remove our shortcomings.

In order to live sanely and grow spiritually as we continue to refrain from compulsive eating one day at a time, we find it best to make the Principles we have learned in Steps Six and Seven a part of our daily lives. We cultivate the willingness to have any newly discovered fears, resentments, and other shortcomings removed. Then, as part of our daily prayer and meditation, we hold these defects up to the light of God's love and humbly ask God to remove them from us, being willing to take any action our Higher Power would have us take.

If we are patient and persistent, we can learn a lot about ourselves and why we feel and act the way we do. We might see that some of our shortcomings are simply misapplied character traits. When applied to the right things at the right times, these same traits that have hurt us so much become great assets. For example, stubbornness is a shortcoming when it keeps us from letting go of self-destructive behaviors. When working a Twelve Step program, however, stubbornness can be an asset. It may be the only thing that keeps us coming back, practicing the Principles, and using the Tools of the program, even when we're slow to see results. In order to "remove" a shortcoming such as stubbornness, our Higher Power might help us to understand it as perseverance and to use it correctly.

Repeated practice of Step Seven enables us to form a working partnership with our Higher Power through which we are relieved of the defects that have blocked our effectiveness in the world. As we gain new humility and ever greater freedom from our character defects, God's power flows more surely and freely through us, bringing healing to others as well as ourselves, and drawing to us all the things we once fought so hard to attain: self-esteem, a feeling of usefulness, joy, strength to surmount difficulties, fellowship, and love. Our simple prayers, humbly spoken, are answered in wonderful ways as we open our lives to God's transforming power, and we find that, once again, God does for us what we could never do for ourselves.

# STEP EIGHT

Made a list of all persons we had harmed and
became willing to make amends to them all.

---

In our days of out-of-control eating and food behaviors, most of us were so obsessed with food we had little time to develop or nurture effective relationships with other people. When we were eating compulsively, we may not have fully realized how we had isolated ourselves. We may have felt that once the food problem was solved, everything in our lives would be satisfactory. When we did stop eating compulsively, however, we usually found that our defective ways of dealing with others were a source of pain for us. In many cases, this pain was so great we were tempted to eat again rather than face it. "What's the use of abstaining if I'm just going to hurt?" we asked. "If this is recovery, I don't want it!" Clearly, if we were going to remain abstinent and find serenity, we had to learn better ways of dealing with other people, ways that would bring us joy instead of pain. Step Eight is designed to help us with this process. In Step Eight, we look at our relationships for the purpose of discovering those patterns that have done harm to us and others. Here, we meet guilt head-on and get rid of it. We learn about the healing power of forgiveness as we discover how to forgive ourselves and others. Most important, we begin to become willing to make *amends*—that is, to make *changes*—in the way we deal with the people who share our lives.

Step Eight is a two-part process, the first part is to write a list of all persons we have harmed. In deciding whom to include on the list, we may have some trouble determining what actually is harmful to others. Oddly enough, the question of how to identify harm rarely arises when we're remembering the harm done to us. We know very well what actions by others have caused *us* harm! Perhaps to help us answer the question of "what is harm," we might think about some of the ways we've been hurt and ask ourselves, "Have I ever dealt with another person in a similar way?" When we answer this question honestly, we may be surprised to learn that we ourselves have given others the same sort of treatment that hurt us the most when we were on the receiving end.

The written moral inventory we did in Step Four can help us to make a list of those we have harmed. As we work Step Eight, we look back over what we wrote on our Fourth Step, and we draw from that inventory a list of names, adding to this list any others we have harmed. If we have lost or destroyed our Fourth Step inventory, the questions in the Step Four chapter of this book can be used in making our Eighth Step list. We go over these questions carefully, paying close attention to those that deal with ways in which our character defects have affected other people.

Many of us have found that our own name belongs somewhere near the top of our Eighth Step list. Yes, we have harmed others, but we have also damaged ourselves with our self-destructive thinking, eating, and living habits. We have learned that a complete willingness to make amends to ourselves and to forgive ourselves for past mistakes has been essential to our recovery.

We need to include the names of all those we can remember having harmed, even the ones who hurt us first. It doesn't matter how badly some of these people may have treated us; we now look with complete honesty at our side of each relationship. If we did those individuals any harm at all, we need to list them and the harm we did. It might help us to remember that our purpose in doing Step Eight is not to judge others, but to learn attitudes of mercy and forgiveness.

However, we might mistakenly go to the other extreme and put on the list names that don't belong there. If someone hurt us or was rude to us and we feel badly toward that person, we can begin to heal this situation through forgiveness. That individual's name does not need to appear on our amends list unless we have also harmed him or her in some way. We're not doing Step Eight to make others feel better or like us more, we're doing it for ourselves, so that *we* can recover. In cases about which we're confused, our sponsors can help us sort out whom we have and have not harmed.

Once we have gone back through our lives and are sure that we have written down the names of all those we have harmed, we are ready to work the second half of Step Eight. Now our task is more difficult: We must become willing to make amends to all those on our list. In many cases, this can seem like a frightening and humiliating prospect. We know we have done wrong and are sorry, but to actually confess our deeds to the very people we've wronged seems impossible. After years of running from any kind of unpleasantness and hiding ourselves in food so we wouldn't have to feel embarrassment or pain, we're now asked to admit our mistakes and face all their consequences. We're asked to do so while being abstinent, without eating compulsively to numb our feelings. How can we possibly become willing?

Our sponsors and other OA members who have walked this way before us can have good suggestions to help us with this task of becoming willing. At this stage of the program more than at any other, we should not try to go it alone. Here, we have found it best to take our amends list to our sponsor and discuss the various problems with her or him. First of all, an experienced OA member is able to help us by making sure we actually do owe amends in each case. Further, a sponsor's suggestions about how to go about making amends can help us to become willing. As we frankly discuss the actions we might take and words we might say, the making of amends begins to seem less threatening. For the first time, we begin to feel that we really may be able to face the people we have harmed.

Our sponsors often encourage us to think about forgiveness as we work through Step Eight. As long as we have not forgiven people for harms they have done to us, we will find it impossible to make sincere amends to them for our side of the conflicts. Even in cases where we manage to find the willingness to talk to them, we're very likely to bring up their mistakes and wind up insulting them, rather than to make amends. Even if we don't bring up their mistakes directly, our ill will toward them will come through in other ways, if we have not truly forgiven them.

We need to forgive ourselves for what we regret doing or not doing, and for not being all we could have been. Self-forgiveness means letting go of negative feelings, such as shame and guilt. The power to extend forgiveness to others comes from self-forgiveness. To refuse to forgive is to continue to hurt ourselves. Forgiveness is not forgetting or pretending something didn't happen. We acknowledge that we were harmed, but we need to let go of the pain in order to move forward with our recovery. Forgiveness is not excusing: A wrong was, in fact, committed. Forgiveness is not giving permission for the hurtful behavior to continue or saying the behavior in the past was okay. Nor is forgiveness necessarily reconciliation. That is a separate decision.

Since forgiveness is essential to completing Step Eight, some discussion of how to forgive another person is in order. Many of us have been told all our lives that we ought to forgive those who wrong us, but rarely have we been taught how to do so.

Our first step toward forgiving someone, oddly enough, might be to write down the reasons why we are angry with this person. The writing process can be very healing because, more than any other

Tool of our program, it gets us in touch with our true feelings. Writing clarifies emotions that have been confused and buried in us, sometimes for many years. Also, by writing down our grievances, we place a boundary around them. Whether the writing of them takes up two paragraphs or twenty pages, whether it takes us minutes or hours, we finally see there is a limit to how much we have been hurt. Our grievances are only so big and no bigger. The hurt had a beginning, and it can have an end as well.

Often, after writing down our feelings, we find it helpful to give away what we've written in some way. Perhaps we will want to read it to a sponsor or another person not involved in the hurtful situation. Perhaps we will want to put it away for a week or so, then get it out and read it again ourselves. Often when we do this, we find that we are already feeling better about the situation, that our pain is not as great as when we first wrote it down. Finally, we may want to symbolically release the hurt, perhaps by burning the writing or tearing up the paper we have written on and throwing the pieces away.

If we still have bad feelings toward the person who has harmed us, we might try prayer as a powerful technique for ridding ourselves of the resentment. People with long experience in living by the Twelve Steps have found that prayer can bring the ability to forgive even the most devastating wrongs. If we pray daily for the people who have wronged us, asking that they be given all that we want for ourselves, we can be freed of our resentments and forgive them for the harm they have done to us. The action of praying for those we resent will work, even if we don't mean a word of what we're saying. If we keep praying for them faithfully, sooner or later our feelings will change. When our feelings change, when we find ourselves being sincere in asking God to bless the people we have resented, then we will know we have forgiven them. Like much of our program of recovery, forgiveness is an ongoing practice. We may feel our resentment toward an individual resurface at times. For some of our more troubling issues, we may need to repeat these measures in order to maintain our serenity.

After we forgive those who have hurt us, we are much more willing to make amends. This does not mean we will suddenly want to go through with this ego-puncturing process. We are not likely to be eager to face the people we've harmed and frankly discuss our mistakes with them. We need to remember, however, that we can be *willing* to do something we don't *want* to do.

As much as we might like to, we cannot skip the making of amends if we want freedom from compulsive eating. The experience of OA members who have worked the Steps before us shows that recovery depends on completing Steps Eight and Nine. With this in mind, we turn once more to God, asking for the willingness to do the things we fear, to make the amends we owe. Having said this prayer sincerely, we are now willing, and we move quickly ahead to Step Nine.

# STEP NINE

Made direct amends to such people wherever possible,
except when to do so would injure them or others.

---

*SPIRITUAL PRINCIPLE*

## LOVE

For many members of Overeaters Anonymous, Step Nine proves to be the most surprising of the Twelve. Before we do the Step, most of us dread the thought of going to each person we've harmed, frankly acknowledging our faults, and taking direct action to remedy the damage we have done or repay the losses we have caused. After making amends, however, those of us who dreaded Step Nine the most are eager to share the results. This Step has freed us from the shackles of our past mistakes in a miraculous way. Our lives are changed, our broken relationships mended, and the resentment that poisoned our hearts for years is washed away.

Those of us still facing Step Nine may have heard about the benefits of making amends from those who've already done this Step. Even so, our fears might make us want to procrastinate. We're warned that to put off making our amends would immobilize us and threaten our recovery from compulsive eating and destructive food behaviors. As soon as we become willing in Step Eight, we need to move ahead quickly and act on that willingness.

We also need to exercise common sense as we set about this process. The Ninth Step specifically warns us of the danger of doing more harm than good as we face people directly and talk with them about hurtful situations of the past. For this reason, many of us have found it advisable to discuss the actions we are about to take with another person who has already taken the Step, an adviser who has personal experience with the Twelve Step way of life or preferably our sponsors. We have probably already discussed some of our plans in the process of becoming willing to make amends. Now we need to resolve any lingering questions and doubts about how we should proceed. We do this by checking our words and actions ahead of time with someone more experienced, someone who is detached from the situation.

Our sponsors may remind us the purpose of Step Nine is to clear away guilt and ill will that stands in the way of establishing better relationships with people whom our lives have touched. In most cases, this requires us to do more than just say "I'm sorry." In making amends, we need to acknowledge the specific harm we've done, apologize, make appropriate restitution, and change our behavior toward them in the future.

Before starting out to make amends, we must let go of any expectations of how others will receive us. In most cases, we'll be treated better than we've anticipated. Sometimes people won't even remember that we ever harmed them. Others might refuse our attempts to make restitution. In some rare instances, there will be those who refuse to accept our apologies. If this happens, we release these people with love. We cannot control how others receive our amends. They have the right to hold grudges against us the rest of their lives if they choose to. They don't owe us forgiveness, and we don't need their forgiveness to complete Step Nine and recover from compulsive eating. Our only job is to clear off our side of the street by doing whatever we can to right our wrongs. Having done so, we no longer need to feel any guilt or anger about these situations.

Clearing off our side of the street requires us to be sincere and direct in our approach to the people we've hurt. We may be tempted to spare ourselves embarrassment by making some vague statement about being sorry for any harm we may have done. In a few cases, this is the most appropriate way to make amends. Most of the time, however, a loosely worded apology does not show true sincerity on our part. We need to remember that we owe the victims of our wrong actions an honest and straightforward acknowledgment of our mistakes.

At the same time, we would usually do well to keep the wording of our apologies as simple as possible, in order to avoid dragging in facts and details that might hurt people all over again. Certainly, we should avoid mention of things they may have done to provoke us, even if we feel those things are much worse than our own mistakes. Having forgiven these people in Step Eight, we now stick to a simply worded statement of the things *we* did to cause *them* harm, and we express our sincere regrets. We avoid excuses, dramatizations, or a detailed rehashing of events surrounding our actions.

We might say something like this: "Mrs. Jones, I stole money from your drawer several times when I was working for you last summer. I'm very sorry for the losses you suffered due to my dishonesty." Or: "John, I realize that I made a habit of belittling you, and I want to apologize. It was wrong of me to treat you that way."

In most cases, we would do well to go ahead and tell the people to whom we're making the amends what sorts of changes or restitutions we are undertaking, making clear we are glad for a chance to set right our wrongs. If we have physically or materially harmed anyone, if we have stolen or damaged property, or if we have cost anyone money by our actions, we should pay or make arrangements to pay the money we owe. If we have lied to someone or about someone, we should now set the record straight, providing we can do so without causing further harm.

To amend something means to change it. We complete our

amends for our wrongful actions of the past by changing our actions in the future. This is especially important when making amends to ourselves and those people close to us whom we have repeatedly harmed by our patterns of behavior. We owe such people "living amends." The words we say to them are not nearly so important as how we act toward them from now on. Were we to apologize, but then go right on hurting them, our words would be empty indeed, and a real improvement in our damaged relationships would be unlikely. Only by permanently changing our harmful attitudes and actions can we make it up to ourselves and our loved ones for the hurts of the past.

These, then, are the actions we take to make direct amends in each case where it is possible. However, there may be some people on our amends list whom we cannot find. Although direct amends to such people are impossible right now, we can begin by making indirect amends to them. For instance, we might put in writing the words we would say to them if we could see them face-to-face. We might write down our acknowledgement of the wrong we did and outline our plans to make things right with them. As we go on with our program, we'll need to continue searching for them, resolving to make the amends directly once we've found them. We are sometimes surprised by the sudden reappearance of people on our amends list who have been out of our lives for years.

Some of the people on our Eighth Step list may have died, so we cannot make direct amends to them. We've found it is healing for us to go ahead and make these amends indirectly. Again, we could begin by writing down the words we would say to them if they were alive. Then we might read the letter out loud at some place that reminds us of them. The restitution part of our amends might be made by giving a gift to their favorite charity, helping a member of their family, or in some other appropriate manner.

Appropriateness is our guide each time we make amends, whether we make them directly or indirectly. Some amends fall in the category of those that we cannot make directly without harming somebody. For instance, to go to the spouse of someone with whom we've had an affair and confess could be very harmful, unless we're sure this person already knows about the affair. It also helps us to remember that we make direct amends for our *actions* (or inaction when action was called for) rather than for our *feelings*. To go to someone and say "I'm sorry I've disliked you all these years" is inappropriate and will only inflict pain. The appropriate way to make up for five years of secret jealousy or hatred is to replace it with five years of open acceptance, respect, and love.

Some amends may need to be made anonymously to avoid hurting innocent people. However, we don't make our amends anonymously simply to avoid embarrassment to ourselves, nor do we rationalize that making amends would injure *us* financially or damage *our* self-esteem. Were we to skip doing some of our amends, we would deprive ourselves of the full healing and freedom that comes when we work the Ninth Step thoroughly, and so we'd be hurting ourselves rather than doing ourselves a favor.

If we are to be restored to right relations with others, we must do whatever we can to square things with the people we have harmed. Much of what we need to do to make amends won't be easy, but those who have gone through with Step Nine have always found it to be more than worth the effort. When we finish our amends most of us feel closer to our Higher Power than ever before.

As we have dealt lovingly with every person in our lives, our spiritual awakening has become a reality. To the best of our ability, we've cleaned up the wreckage of the past, and we are more at peace with the world.

Now that we have completed the first nine Steps, we can face the future with a new confidence. We no longer need the crutch of excess food because we have discovered a way of life that nourishes us physically, emotionally, and spiritually. Our challenge from here on will be to continue following this path daily as we are guided by the last three Steps of our Twelve Step program.

# STEP TEN

Continued to take personal inventory and when we were wrong, promptly admitted it.

---

*SPIRITUAL PRINCIPLE*

## PERSEVERANCE

**M**any of us have come to Overeaters Anonymous after years of pursuing short-term solutions to our long- term problem of compulsive eating. One aspect of this program that keeps us here is the promise of permanent recovery from this baffling disease. But what in this world is truly permanent? We read on page 204 of our *For Today* book, "Repetition is the only form of permanence that nature can achieve."[6] If we are to experience permanent recovery from compulsive overeating, we will have to repeat, day after day, the actions that have already brought us so much healing.

Through the first nine Steps of our program, we have made a beginning on an entirely new way of life, one of sane eating and

---

[6] *For Today* (Overeaters Anonymous, Inc., © 1982) p. 204.

successful living. Step Ten calls for daily repetition of the actions we took in the first nine Steps. As we do so, these actions become patterns for us to follow in the future—patterns that will enable us to thrive, grow spiritually, and be happy without excess food or compulsive food behaviors.

The Tenth Step begins with the word "continued," our first clue that perseverance is about to become a key aspect of our recovery program. In the past, we may have clung stubbornly to self-destructive eating and other harmful behaviors. Now we need to be stubborn about working our program, even during those times when we feel as though it isn't working or we aren't recovering quickly enough. Stubbornness turned to such good use becomes perseverance as we continue—day after day—to apply to our lives the same Principles we learned in Steps Four through Nine.

In Step Four, for instance, we learned to take a personal moral inventory, look honestly and fearlessly at ourselves, and recognize our liabilities and assets. Step Ten asks us to continue this practice daily. The purpose of Step Ten is to identify and remove from our path today's stumbling blocks, those manifestations of pride, fear, anger, self-pity, greed, and other emotions that are bringing pain into our lives and keeping us from growing today. We have found that all of us inevitably encounter these feelings, and it only makes matters worse if we deny we have them or try to will them away. Step Ten allows us to recognize our emotions and walk through the pain they cause us. We then let them go, turning our feelings over to our Higher Power so that we can regain our emotional balance.

In Steps Five through Nine we ventured outside of our isolation to share ourselves in depth with our Higher Power and with other people. Most of us had spent our lives before OA trying to go it alone. As we worked these Steps, we learned how much healing and help there is in loving connections with a Power greater than ourselves and those who share our lives. We now want to continue strengthening these connections, and we have a way to do that through our practice of Step Ten.

There are many ways to take a personal inventory. The simplest is taken mentally, and some veterans in the Twelve Step way of life have become so adept at this practice that self-analysis is second nature. A spot-check inventory, taken whenever we find ourselves facing difficulties, is something we can learn to do in a few moments of quiet reflection whenever the need arises. With practice, it becomes easier to recognize the exact nature of our problems and see what actions we need to take to restore our serenity, actions we will want to carry out "promptly," as Step Ten advises. Perhaps we've forgotten our Step Three decision and are trying to control some aspect of our lives by self-will. Do we need to discuss the problem with our sponsors, or ask our Higher Power to remove a character defect? Have we wronged someone and now owe amends? Are we applying the Twelve Steps and their underlying Principles to our situation? Once we begin to practice this pattern of on-the-spot analysis and action whenever we're disturbed, it becomes a habit for us, and we discover we've learned an amazing new set of skills for successful living.

When something more than a spot-check is called for, many of us have found it helpful to write our Step Ten inventory. Putting our thoughts and feelings down on paper or describing a troubling incident helps us to better understand our actions and reactions in a way that is often not revealed to us by simply thinking or talking about them. When we write about our difficulties, it becomes easier to see situations more clearly and perhaps better discern any actions that need to be taken.

Some of us make a daily habit of reviewing our emotions and behavior of the past twenty-four hours. A more leisurely and careful analysis than the spot-check inventory, a daily inventory may be written or done mentally. Its purpose is to reveal those areas where we're having difficulties in our daily lives and help us determine what we can do about them. It also serves as a reminder of those things that are going well for us and for which we are grateful. There are several ways to take a daily inventory. Some of us simply review the major events of the day in chronological order, making note of the feelings we had and how we dealt with those feelings. Some of us draw up a balance sheet, listing negative feelings and events on one side, and positive feelings and events on the other. Some of us work from a list of common character defects and assets, such as fear/faith, resentment/acceptance, greed/generosity, and so on. Referring to this list, we ask ourselves such questions as: "What fears did I experience today, and how did I react to them?" Then we list or recall those instances when we became aware that our former defects had been removed; when we acted on faith; when we were accepting and forgiving, letting go of resentments; when we were selfless; or when we exhibited other positive character traits.

In taking daily inventory, we seek to become increasingly aware of our true motives and emotions. We seek to examine our actions, in particular to identify where we were resentful, dishonest, fearful, self-seeking, and inconsiderate, so we can learn from our mistakes and build on our successes. Our purpose is not to stir up negative feelings and guilt, but to continue along the path of progress and to recognize those areas of our lives where progress is being made. After we have taken our daily inventory, we can follow through with the second half of Step Ten, which says, "when we were wrong, promptly admitted it." This simple little clause implies that we have the opportunity to do more than just look at our defects and assets. We can take the same actions with them that we did with the character traits we found in our Fourth Step inventory: discuss them with our Higher Power, sponsors, or, perhaps, another person; turn the defects over, asking our Higher Power to remove them; and make amends where they are due. Some OA members connect with their sponsors daily to review their Tenth Step inventory. We discuss our problems and successes with our Higher Power in prayer as well, daily asking for help to let go of defects and expressing gratitude when we discover that defects are removed and problems resolved. Inevitably, there are those times when we make mistakes and harm other people. Step Ten tells us that we make amends *promptly,* as soon as we realize someone has been harmed. By doing this, we bring a new honesty into our relationships. We find we can save ourselves days of resentment and fear by resolving disputes as they arise, instead of allowing wounds to fester.

A Tenth Step inventory can also be more extensive, similar to the one we took in Step Four but dealing with problems we may not have been aware of when we originally took the Fourth Step. A need to re-inventory some aspects of our past does not mean we failed to do Step Four properly. It simply shows that we have grown in self-awareness and have become ready to face and resolve aspects of our lives that we were not capable of dealing with the first time around. Each of us is an individual with individual needs, and no two of us proceed at exactly the same pace or work this program in exactly the same way.

An extensive Tenth Step inventory might focus on one particular character defect, behavior pattern, or area of life. We will probably want to write this inventory, as we did the Fourth Step, and we will certainly want to follow through with prompt action. As soon as possible, we will want to give this inventory away to another person. After that, we will repeat the actions of Steps Six and Seven, asking our Higher Power to heal our wounds, remove any defects we have discovered in our investigation, and help us change our behavior. Then we'll complete this course of action by listing and making any amends we might owe in connection with events listed in this inventory.

A persistent effort to let go of our defects and change our actions is crucial to our recovery from here on. As we become aware of shortcomings through the inventory process, there are several actions we can take to be rid of them. One such action is to imagine how we might behave if we did not have a particular defect. We could picture ourselves in the circumstances where we have acted out our shortcoming, but see ourselves acting differently this time. Anything we can imagine, we can do, with the help of our Higher Power. We might even speak the new words or act out the improved set of behaviors, just for practice. Through this kind of action, we daily affirm to ourselves that we can change and are changing, with God's help. At first, we may slip back into the old ways in moments of pressure, but we won't let this discourage us. We've spent a lifetime learning to do things the old ways, so of course the old behaviors feel much more natural to us. As time goes on, however, God helps us to let go of our defects and replace them with positive thoughts and actions. God will, that is, if we persist in doing whatever we can to change.

As with the Fourth Step inventory, the Tenth Step inventory may uncover aspects of our past with which we need professional help. Our OA friends are sympathetic and loving, but few are trained to recognize and deal with deeply rooted psychological problems, and OA is not the place to seek such help.

As we repeatedly act on Step Ten, we begin to see the remarkable way the Steps can, from now on, continue to remove unnecessary turmoil and pain from our lives. The new attitudes of honesty about our problems and surrender to a Power greater than ourselves have become a part of us by now; they are the basis of every choice we make in our day-to-day lives. Reviewing our recent behavior, keeping our Higher Power in charge of our lives, asking for guidance, and promptly admitting our errors, becomes a sane and satisfying way of life—far better than nursing our fears or building a fresh set of resentments to harbor. Forced to adopt this new way of coping with life in order to recover from compulsive eating, we now find ourselves grateful for this program in its own right. Practicing the program has given us many gifts—gifts that we wouldn't trade for the quick-and-easy solutions to our compulsive overeating many of us once sought in every new diet. More gifts are in store for us as we continue working the program and experiencing the miracle of permanent recovery, one day at a time.

# STEP ELEVEN

Sought through prayer and meditation to improve our conscious contact with God *as we understood Him,* praying only for knowledge of His will for us and the power to carry that out.

---

*SPIRITUAL PRINCIPLE*
### SPIRITUAL AWARENESS

When we began attending Overeaters Anonymous meetings, most of us were attracted by the unconditional acceptance we experienced here. That life-changing acceptance has continued to sustain us as we've worked the Steps and faced the changes that have come about in our lives as a result. Now, as we encounter Step Eleven, we are challenged to seek out more direct conscious contact with the ultimate source of that life-changing love.

In OA, we share a belief that we can each recover through a spiritual relationship with a Power that is greater than ourselves alone. While based on this shared belief, our program does not promote or favor any particular concept of the exact nature of this Power. In OA meetings, we often hear the power source called "my Higher Power" or, more succinctly, "HP." This can be disconcerting to newcomers, but for those who've been around long enough to work through the first ten Steps, the term "Higher Power" signals a freedom we've come to appreciate and even treasure—the freedom to encounter this healing force directly and express our beliefs however we choose. In order to recover from compulsive eating and other compulsive food behaviors, we need an ongoing relationship with this Higher Power, and we find having complete freedom to seek that relationship is a vital aspect of our program.

It takes more than spiritual freedom, however, to establish and develop a relationship with a Power greater than ourselves. We have to take action. In Step Eleven, we are challenged to actively seek to improve our relationship with our Higher Power in the same way we might develop any relationship, by taking the time on a regular basis to be with HP. Most of us have found it necessary to set aside some time each day when we can be alone and undisturbed. During this time, we can actively seek to develop a consciousness of our power source through prayer and meditation, and to do so with an attitude of complete trust, asking only for knowledge of God's will for us and the power to carry it out.

We may feel awkward about regular daily prayer at first. Step Eleven encourages us to *practice* prayer, to continue talking to our Higher Power daily, even when it seems like a senseless exercise. When we have committed to Step Eleven, giving a part of each day to meditation and prayer consistently, we have been rewarded—and sometimes awed—by the results. For many of us, a regular daily quiet time for prayer and meditation is essential, a part of this program we don't want to live without, for it gives us the direction and strength we need to live the rest of that day effectively. Many of us begin and end our day with prayer and meditation and also use these practices at all times during the day when we feel the need for guidance, strength, or serenity.

Step Eleven is not intended to interfere with or replace the traditional religious practices some of us follow. Rather, we have found that this enhances the practice of our chosen religion. At the same time, neither Step Eleven nor any other Step requires us to adopt an organized religion.

As with so many other aspects of this program, there is no one right way to do Step Eleven. "Keep it simple" is a good slogan to apply here. Remembering that our goal is to develop a closer conscious contact with God, prayer is simply what we do when we talk with our Higher Power, and meditation is simply a way of stilling our minds, listening, and opening our spirits to God's influence.

What do we say when we talk with God? We say whatever we feel like saying. Some of us begin to practice prayer by reciting prayers we have memorized, read in program literature or other books, learned in meetings, or remember from childhood. There are many wonderful prayers available, which over the centuries have nourished those seeking spiritual growth. As we say these prayers day after day and think about their meaning for us in our present circumstances, we are beginning to practice meditation as well, though we may not realize it. As we fix our attention on the truths contained in these prayers, we open our minds to receive new understanding and direction from our Higher Power.

In addition to repeating memorized prayers, we can express ourselves to God in our own words, much as we might talk with our best friend. Some of us have been taught that there are things we shouldn't say to God or feelings we shouldn't express. However, now that we're recovering from compulsive eating, we need complete freedom to express our honest feelings in any situation, without fear of saying the wrong thing and damaging or destroying our relationship with God. Such freedom is an essential factor in the healing process because recovery is based on the practice of honesty with ourselves and our Higher Power. We need the security that comes from knowing that nothing can destroy our relationship with this all-important source of healing and strength while we honestly explore our deepest selves.

The Eleventh Step guides us to ask only for knowledge of God's will for us and the power to carry that out. Since we have turned our will and lives over to the care of this Higher Power, it makes little sense for us to spend our prayer time giving God instructions. Does this mean we are never to discuss our needs and problems in prayer, never to express our feelings, fears, or desires? Clearly, if we are to develop a vital relationship with a Higher Power, we need to bring into our prayers all the things that concern us. We pray about these things, not so we can get our way, but so we can bring our will regarding them into alignment with God's will.

All of us who seek to develop a relationship with a Higher Power through prayer experience times when we feel angry with God. Perhaps in the past our reaction to this anger has been to pretend it didn't exist, denying our anger to God and to ourselves. Or perhaps we reacted by giving up on prayer entirely. As we seek to recover with God's help, neither of those options work for us any longer. So we go ahead and express our anger, but we keep on talking to God. The anger passes, answers come, and we find that we have drawn closer to our Higher Power through this experience.

Many of us have found that the practice of writing down our angry feelings or other concerns in letters to God is a great help. As we write, we clarify issues, we express our feelings honestly, and we communicate with our Higher Power in a way that is very tangible to us. OA members have been known to deliver prayer letters to God in all sorts of ways. We've mailed them to our sponsors, put them in a can we've labeled our "God can," or disposed of them in other ways that symbolized our letting go. Such private rituals often seemed silly to us at first, but we've found they work wonders. The key is that we've stopped worrying, taken an action, and turned our problems over to our Higher Power. Our energies are no longer bound up in our worries and resentments, and we are free to move forward again, to do God's will.

Meditation is our way of quieting our minds so we can get better acquainted with this Higher Power of ours. As with prayer, there is no one right way to practice meditation; in fact, most of us vary our practice from time to time. The only way to do meditation wrong is not to do it at all. We compulsive people are oriented to action. Meditation is an action that gives us much-needed practice in the art of sitting still and opening our hearts to receive spiritual nourishment. Many of us have spent a lot of time running—running from the food, then running to it—and many of us have turned to excess food for its sedative effect. Eating compulsively was our chief means of relaxation. Meditation offers us a way to stop running and to relax without eating compulsively.

When meditating, we consciously choose to focus our minds on something other than our everyday desires and concerns. We might begin to do this by breathing deeply and counting our breaths, by holding a special object and concentrating on how it feels, by listening to soft music, by repeating a word or phrase, by concentrating on an image, by staring at an object or picture, or by other means. When we are distracted by worries or annoyances, we practice gently letting go of these distractions and returning our attention to listening to what our Higher Power has to tell us. Our purpose in meditating is simple: We seek to relax and receive spiritual nourishment by experiencing more fully our connections with our true unfragmented selves and with our Higher Power.

Step Eleven implies that through our practice of prayer and meditation we will come to know God's will for us. Here the question arises: How, exactly, are we to know which thoughts are God's directions and which are our own rationalizations? A communication from God might be difficult for us to recognize at first because it probably won't come in audible words. Instead, it may come in the form of a new idea or concept, it may come as a change in our motives or attitudes, or it may simply be a feeling we have that our energy has been renewed or our bad mood has lifted. We can recognize a communication from our Higher Power by the effect it has on us. If time spent in prayer and meditation makes us even a little bit saner or more loving, if it encourages or strengthens us even a tiny bit, we can be sure God has "spoken" and we have "heard."

Our sponsors and other OA members with experience in prayer and meditation can also help us recognize God's direction. When we believe we have received insight from our Higher Power, we find it wise to discuss the matter with our sponsors or spiritual advisors before we take any drastic action. There may be times when we're faced with an important decision and want to know our Higher Power's will. Our sponsors or OA friends might suggest that we pray about it, asking God to increase our desire to take the action if we are supposed to take it, or decrease our desire if we're not supposed to take it. After this prayer, we stop worrying about making the decision right now and we wait a day or so, meanwhile keeping our eyes, ears, and minds open. By the end of the waiting period, we will inevitably find that we've gained a clearer perspective on the decision. Despite our most sincere efforts, we sometimes make an error in acting on what we think is God's will for us. In time, we may be grateful for the lessons we have learned in these situations. It is through such experiences that we grow more adept at recognizing the will of our Higher Power in the future.

OA members who have made prayer and meditation a regular part of their lives have found a resource for healing and strength that cannot fail. Sponsors, OA friends, meetings, and literature are wonderful sources of help for us. We wouldn't want to be without any of these resources because we often find God speaks to us through them. From time to time, however, we may not have access to them in a moment of need. Our Higher Power is the only source of help that is always available to us, always strong enough to lift us up and set our feet on the path of life. Prayer and meditation are our links to this unfailing source. Practiced regularly, they open our lives to the comfort we sought in food but could never find. Through prayer and meditation, we align ourselves with a Higher spiritual Power that gives us everything we need to live to our fullest potential.

# STEP TWELVE

Having had a spiritual awakening as the result of
these Steps, we tried to carry this message to
compulsive overeaters and to practice these principles
in all our affairs.

---

*SPIRITUAL PRINCIPLE*

**SERVICE**

S tep Twelve begins with the acknowledgment of a great truth:
We who have worked the first eleven Steps of the Overeaters
Anonymous program have had a spiritual awakening, and we now
have a message of hope to carry to other compulsive overeaters.
We who once suffered from complete powerlessness to control our
eating and our lives have now discovered the saving strength of a
Power greater than ourselves. We have experienced the miracle of
physical, emotional, and spiritual healing, just as we were promised
when we began working these Steps.

For most of us, the central factor in this spiritual awakening has been our decision to trust a Higher Power with every aspect of our lives. In acting on that decision, one day at a time, we have learned a whole new set of skills for living, skills that enable us to clear from our lives everything that might interfere with our trust in this Higher Power. Now we know we don't have to fear anything that comes to us. Even when challenges happen, as they do in life, we know we have a way of sanely facing each situation. We have seen that our Higher Power will reveal something of value to us with every experience, as long as we continue practicing these spiritual Principles.

We're no longer afraid of food because it no longer controls us. The glorious fact for most of us is that God has lifted the food obsession from us. Freed of the obsession and restored to sanity, today we choose not to eat self-destructively. We have new ways of coping with our problems and new practices now, which make living a positive, joyful experience most of the time. If we should again crave more food than we need, we know we can find relief in the Steps instead of in compulsive eating.

This being true, are we now ready to complete the Twelfth Step and graduate from OA? Looking back at how far we've come, many of us have been tempted to think we've arrived at the end of the journey. The truth, learned from the experiences of thousands of OA members, is that, no matter how great our physical, emotional, and spiritual transformation, we still aren't cured. This is true even when we've reached the goal of a healthy body weight, even when we've worked all Twelve Steps to the best of our ability, even when we've celebrated milestone anniversaries of abstinence and recovery, even when we've been placed in positions of trust by other OA members and have rendered service to our groups and service bodies. The Twelfth Step invites us to continue the journey one day at a time for the rest of our lives. We need to keep moving forward in recovery, keep developing our spiritual consciousness, if we are to remain spiritually awake and fully alive. Perhaps it is fortunate for us, and for the millions of compulsive overeaters who still suffer, that most of us who've worked this program will be unable to keep the recovery we have unless we share our experience, strength, and hope with others. Some of us have tried to follow our program in isolation and have been unable to keep our emotional balance and abstinence. Had this been possible, we might not be here today to carry the message to those who still suffer. We would have missed the best part of the Twelve Steps, for the greatest joy of recovery comes to us when we share our OA program with others.

Few of us suspected this would be so when we started working the Steps. For years, we've looked for gratification in unbridled eating; in material possessions; in careers; in our many attempts to have perfect bodies; and in money, sex, and social status. Although most of us have received and enjoyed some of these things, the satisfaction we felt in them was small compared with the joy we have found in sharing this program with other compulsive overeaters.

Helping other compulsive eaters through sponsoring and other forms of service to our groups, service bodies, and OA as a whole has been a surprisingly powerful factor in our recovery. Simple actions that seemed unimportant when we took them have turned out to have profound effects on us and on others. Hugs we've given at meetings, phone calls we've made, letters we've written, simple words of encouragement we've spoken and quickly forgotten have come back to us—sometimes at the very moment we've needed them most—from people who received through them the strength to continue their journey of recovery. Most of us who have been around OA for more than a few months have seen miracles of recovery in our meetings. We count among our friends people whom we first met when they were suffering newcomers. We've seen them transformed by this simple program, and we are gratified to have played our part, even if all we did was show up at OA meetings and say, "Keep coming back!" The joy we receive as we try to carry the message is a positive force in our lives today, sustaining us through good times and hard times, transforming us and our companions in recovery.

Talking about OA with those who still suffer has become an increasingly natural thing for us to do. Sometimes because of the changes in our bodies, and sometimes because of the changes in our attitudes, people now say to us, "You look wonderful! What have you done?" It becomes easier and easier to mention our involvement in OA, to share more of what we've experienced here, to invite other sufferers to join us.

We usually ask God to help us in talking about the program with people outside of OA and with those in meetings. When we turn ourselves over to our Higher Power, we can relax and speak honestly without worrying that we might not say the right thing. Also, we've found it less confusing to others if we make it a habit when sharing about the program to concentrate on our OA experience, rather than on aspects of our experience not related to OA. Though we may have been helped by therapies, church attendance, food plans, exercise programs, self-help books, metaphysics, and the like, we've found it best to emphasize our experience with the Twelve Steps, which are the basis of recovery for all of us.

We've also found that helping others has worked best for us when we had no expectations regarding the outcome. When we have set out to fix other people, we have usually failed, despite lavishing long hours on them. Nor do we need to devise plans for saving the whole world in order to work Step Twelve. God finds many ways to help people through us as long as we are willing to do what we can, when we can, and keep ourselves on the path of spiritual progress.

The Twelfth Step suggests that we continue to practice our new way of acting in life "in all our affairs," and the vast experience of recovering compulsive overeaters confirms the importance of this suggestion. As we've worked the first eleven Steps, the Principles embodied in them have begun to replace our old way of life, which centered on self and compulsive eating. In Step Twelve, we confirm that we have turned our backs on the old ways forever. We are moving in a new direction of spiritual growth.

What are some of the Principles inherent in each Step that we are encouraged to practice in all our affairs? In Step One we learned the Principle of *honesty* as we admitted our personal powerlessness over food and the fact that without help we could not successfully manage our own lives. Now we want to continue being honest with ourselves in all our affairs. One important way we practice honesty today is by admitting that we are still compulsive overeaters, that we still need daily help.

In Step Two, we learned *hope* as we came to believe that a Power greater than ourselves could restore us to sanity. This same hope now underlies all our actions. Even in our loneliest hours, we can remind ourselves of the great truth that we are not alone; even in our weakest moments, we can find the strength we need if we believe it is available to us and ask for it.

In Step Three, we learned *faith* as we made the most important decision we had ever made, the decision to trust God—*as we understand God*—with our will and our lives. Practicing the Principle of faith today means that we no longer go through life acting however we feel like acting at any given moment. Instead, we look to our Higher Power for guidance and strength as we face each decision.

In Steps Four and Five, we learned *courage* and *integrity* as we faced the truth about our defects of character. Applying these Principles in all our affairs means we are no longer ruled by a fear of admitting our mistakes. We have the integrity to show the world our true selves. No longer needing to appear perfect, we can live more fully, having the courage to face up to our mistakes and test our strengths in the challenges of life.

In Step Six, we learned more about the necessity of *willingness* as we became entirely ready to let go of our shortcomings. We apply this Principle in many ways now, learning through each day's experience the difference between self-will and a simple willingness to cooperate with the guidance of our Higher Power.

In Step Seven, we began to understand the meaning of *humility.* We practice this Principle today by continuing to let go of status seeking and of thoughts and actions by which we belittled ourselves and others. We try to remain teachable and to humbly trust God for the removal of our shortcomings.

In Steps Eight and Nine, we looked at the damage we had done to others and set about repairing it. Now we apply the same Principles of *self-discipline* and *love* for others to all our actions.

Self-discipline makes us less likely to hurt other people and quicker to make amends when we do.

Practicing the Principle of love, we learn to accept others as they are, not as we would have them be. We're beginning to take this new attitude not just toward other OA members, but also toward people at home, school, work, and in all areas of our lives. Slowly but surely, we find we are establishing the best possible relationship with each person we know.

In Step Ten, we discovered the value of *perseverance* in working the Twelve Steps. Practicing this Principle in all our affairs today means that we continue to do the things that have brought us healing, even though we sometimes wonder if we still need to, or during times we may not want to. Perseverance brings us the reward of continuing, permanent recovery.

In Step Eleven, we learned the Principle of *spiritual awareness* as we turned our attention to the practices of prayer and meditation. We practice this Principle by seeking an awareness of God's presence in all our affairs and continuing to nurture our spiritual connection through prayer and meditation.

The Principle of *service,* which underlies OA's Twelfth Step, can now guide our actions both inside and outside the program. Here, we experience the great truth that when we let go of our need to control people and simply allow our Higher Power to serve others through us we receive an abundance of joy and strength.

We who began working the Steps in order to recover from compulsive eating now find that, through them, we have embarked on a lifelong journey of spiritual growth. From the isolation of food obsession, we have emerged into a new world. Walking hand in hand with fellow OA members and our Higher Power, we are now exploring this world, using the great spiritual Principles embodied in the Twelve Steps as the map to guide our way. We gratefully follow in the footsteps of many others who have walked this way before us, and we're gratified to be making footprints of our own for others to follow.

Those of us who live this program don't simply carry the message; *we are the message.* Each day that we live well, we *are* well, and we embody the joy of recovery, which attracts others who want what we've found in OA. We're always happy to share our secret: the Twelve Steps of Overeaters Anonymous, which empower each of us to live well and be well, one day at a time.

# INTRODUCTION TO
# THE TWELVE TRADITIONS

When we first came to Overeaters Anonymous, we were focused on our own recovery. Most of us took the OA groups we attended and the OA Fellowship as a whole for granted, not thinking much about how they operated and whether they would continue to be there for us in the future. Soon, however, as we left behind our dependence on food, we began to rely on OA. We felt it was our only safe haven, and we reacted with fear any time we thought this Fellowship might be threatened.

Yet we quickly found that we did not need to be afraid for the health of OA. Overeaters Anonymous has Twelve Traditions that are designed to keep our meetings and service bodies on track, functioning in such a way as to nurture the recovery of all compulsive overeaters who seek help in this Fellowship. This study of the Traditions shows how these twelve suggestions have worked to help individuals, groups, and OA as a whole solve problems, thrive, and be effective instruments for carrying the message of recovery to those who still suffer.

We owe a large debt of gratitude to Alcoholics Anonymous for breaking ground in establishing these Traditions and allowing OA to adapt them to our Fellowship. Developed through long and sometimes painful experience, the Twelve Traditions embody spiritual Principles for living. Those who have studied them carefully have found that these Traditions can be applied effectively to all human relationships, both inside and outside OA. With this in mind, we turn our attention to the Traditions, trusting that, as we come to understand them better, we will be better able to keep OA strong and healthy and ourselves spiritually fit in the face of all challenges.

# TRADITION ONE

Our common welfare should come first; personal recovery depends upon OA unity.

---

*SPIRITUAL PRINCIPLE*

## UNITY

We compulsive overeaters have lived much of our lives in isolation. Many of us preferred to be alone so we could eat the way we wanted without interference. Even when we were surrounded by other people, it became progressively difficult for us to connect with them as our obsession with food, body size, and eating grew. Some of us felt like failures whenever we had to ask for help from anyone other than ourselves.

Our desire to live free of compulsive eating has forced us to change these attitudes. Recovery began for most of us when we got out of isolation and into an OA group. Here we discovered we were not alone. As we opened our hearts to other OA members, we found acceptance, a sense of belonging, and unity with other compulsive overeaters that satisfied us in ways food never could.

Many of us would not be alive today if it were not for our OA groups. Here is the only place we have found recovery from the devastating disease of compulsive eating. If we are to continue to live and recover, we must have the continued support of OA groups and the inspiration of our fellow OA members. What's more, we need daily opportunities to be of service to other compulsive overeaters, opportunities the OA group provides.

Thus, the unity of OA is a matter of life and death to us. However, unity isn't always easy to maintain. OA members come from diverse backgrounds, and in meetings, we sometimes encounter people with very different approaches to recovery. Often, our first impulse is to insist they are doing it all wrong. If we as individuals did not value the common welfare of the Fellowship above our own personal viewpoints, OA would soon split into argumentative factions and would lose the strength that comes from our union of many.

In OA meetings, individuals are lovingly guided to keep the needs of the whole group in mind as we share our experience, strength, and hope. Because all OA groups do not follow the same meeting format, there are often reminders about cross talk, length of sharing, or other established guidelines to inform those in attendance of the group conscience. A respect for unity means that individuals keep in mind the rules of the group. We may want to talk for longer than is suggested, or we may feel that we "just have to share" our advice with someone in a meeting. Tradition One tells us to curb those impulses for the sake of the group.

It is suggested that our meeting formats be geared to keep our groups' practices in line with OA Principles. Ideally, OA is a place where every member has ample opportunity to share. We don't try to confront or fix each other. We save the more intimate details of our lives for one-on-one discussions with our sponsors. It is every member's responsibility to protect the OA spirit of unity and mutual support. When it comes our turn to lead an OA meeting, Tradition One makes it our responsibility to lovingly remind members of the group conscience if it is being ignored.

This does not mean that all OA members must agree on every

issue regarding the operation of the Fellowship. Disagreements about the activities of the group arise every day, and we have to find ways of resolving those disagreements without destroying the unity of our Fellowship. Tradition One guides us to give other people's opinions a respectful hearing. We express our own opinions honestly without belittling those who may disagree. As we listen and speak, we keep our minds and hearts open to our Higher Power's will in all matters. After the discussion is over and the group has made a decision, we don't allow any lingering feelings of conflict to divide the group. In OA, we resolve our differences of opinion by considering the welfare of the group as a whole.

Through experience, OA groups have learned the importance of unity. In one city, a difference of opinion divided the intergroup into two factions, each advocating its own concept of recovery. When months of arguments brought no resolution, one faction formed a new intergroup. A short time later, after members on both sides achieved a degree of tranquility, the two intergroups were encouraged to host a region OA convention. Neither intergroup had the resources to do the job alone; they were forced to sit down face-to-face to find a way to work together. Individuals within each faction willing to do this formed a First Tradition Committee, the purpose of which was to find a basis for unity. Changes in attitudes were needed if the two intergroups were to work together to stage the convention. Because they wanted to work together, the members of the committee began by focusing on the principles they could agree on, rather than on their differences, and finally they came up with a single group conscience. In a joint statement, both intergroups recognized the existence of various recovery approaches within the OA Fellowship. Both recognized that a common need brought them together. They stated that manners of working the program were clearly matters of personal or group conscience, and they agreed to refrain from comment or discussion on their differences.

By respecting these guidelines, the two factions found they could indeed work together to stage a successful OA convention. A decade later, neither intergroup had changed its philosophy on how to work the OA program, and yet both were still flourishing, still holding conventions and Unity Day celebrations together, still very active in OA region and world services events. Each supported many strong OA groups where individuals found recovery through OA's Twelve Steps.[7]

Members of the only OA group in a small town had a similar conflict and found their way to unity as well. Meetings were attended by fewer than ten people, and as with many small OA groups, one or two people who had several years in the program kept the meetings going. One night an OA member who had recently moved to town showed up and told a dramatic story about her near death from compulsive eating. She described how she had found OA and how the program and a plan of eating had saved her life.

The OA members were impressed when this woman told them about her weight loss in excess of 100 pounds and were inspired by the light in her eyes and obvious enthusiasm for the program. One person, who was the group's mainstay, however, got nervous when the transferred member talked about her specific plan of eating. The mainstay herself had experienced a miraculous recovery from compulsive overeating, and she believed part of that miracle was that she had been freed from years of compulsive dieting and food planning. She used her discussion time to speak against the transferred member's plan of eating.

Within weeks factions formed around the mainstay and the transferred member, and heated arguments about the use of the plan of eating dominated the meeting. This went on for several months with very hard feelings on both sides.

Then, one night in late summer, the mainstay and the transferred member found themselves the only two people to show up for the weekly OA meeting. After waiting ten minutes for a third person to arrive, they finally agreed to start the meeting with just the two of them. Together they said the Serenity Prayer and began to follow the meeting format. Sitting face-to-face across the table,

---

[7] In the true spirit of OA unity, the two intergroups have joined with a third and formed one united intergroup in their area.

they took turns discussing their experience, strength, and hope. Little by little, their sharing became more honest. The mainstay found herself admitting to the transferred member how much she envied her recovery and how she'd felt upstaged. The transferred member talked with tears in her eyes of how scared she was of relapse, how she'd wanted to start a group like her old home group but hadn't been able to find anybody willing to join her. More than anything, she said, she needed understanding and support. She longed for the mainstay's strength and admired her experience with OA Principles.

Before the meeting was over, the mainstay and transferred member had agreed to sponsor each other. When other group members returned the following week, they found a whole new atmosphere. The transferred member hadn't given up her plan of eating and the mainstay hadn't adopted it. They still had differing goals for their eating, but they now expressed support for each other in reaching those goals. Even more striking was the new note of love and acceptance in their voices when they shared their reasons for sticking with their differing approaches to a plan of eating. When some group members decided to use the plan of eating, the mainstay didn't try to dissuade them. When other people followed the philosophy of the mainstay, the transferred member didn't argue. They had found there was room for more than one approach to recovery in this little group.

Unity does not mean uniformity. In OA, we learn we can disagree with other people on important issues and still be supportive friends. We listen to others with open minds, and we learn to express ourselves without insisting that everyone must do things our way. As we practice these new skills we begin to better understand ourselves and others. It becomes easier to find ways of doing things that meet everybody's needs.

---

**How well do we practice the Principle of unity? We might ask ourselves a few questions about how we act in our OA groups:**

*Is our group dividing into cliques and being indifferent to some members or newcomers?*

*Do we seek to pull together as a group, or are we divisive? Do we discourage gossip? Do we discourage members from taking each others' inventories?*

*Do we focus on our differences or on what we have in common?*

*Are we kind, even to those whose personalities we dislike? Or do we talk about the love of the OA group while acting hostile to some?*

*Do we encourage everybody to give full attention when speakers and others talk during a meeting? Do side conversations or greetings often distract from the OA meeting?*

*Does our group encourage members to speak briefly, or do we allow some to dominate discussions by talking so much that others don't get a chance to speak?*

*Do those leading our meetings allow newcomers to dominate the discussion or interrupt others, or do we help them to be a part of the group right away by explaining the meeting format and guidelines in a kind way?*

*Do we encourage members to use the phone or other forms of digital communication to help one another, not for complaints and gossip?*

*Do we belittle other OA members or groups whose approaches to working the program are different from ours?*

*Do we support OA activities that bring us into contact with other groups? Have we taken the time to learn about OA as a whole? Do we support OA as a whole to the best of our ability?*

*Do we encourage all of our members to share honestly with the group, even when they're going through rough times? Or, do we take the attitude that those who are having trouble shouldn't share?*

*Do we discuss what our meeting can do to better embrace diversity and unity?*[8]

---

[8] The *Unity with Diversity Checklist* (© Overeaters Anonymous, Inc.) was adopted at the 2014 World Service Business Conference and is available as a download at oa.org.

The First Tradition of unity reminds us of an important truth: We are not alone. We are connected to our fellow human beings. Our emotional and spiritual health depends on the health of our relationships. The disease of compulsive eating, which once isolated us, has now led us to OA. Here, in local groups, sponsorship roles, intergroups and service boards, region assemblies, and OA worldwide, we are learning to connect with other people in ways that nurture all of us as we recover together.

# TRADITION TWO

For our group purpose there is but one ultimate authority—a loving God as He may express Himself in our group conscience. Our leaders are but trusted servants; they do not govern.

---

*SPIRITUAL PRINCIPLE*

**TRUST**

The newcomer may ask, "Who is the head of OA?" and be puzzled by the answer in Tradition Two: a loving God as expressed in the group conscience. The Second Tradition of Overeaters Anonymous may seem thoroughly impractical, but it works. When faced with a problem or challenge, we ask for God's guidance to show us what is best for the group as a whole. Then we discuss the matter carefully, we vote on alternatives, and we trust that the decision we reach together is our Higher Power's will.

Most organizations have a power structure, and as a result, people struggle to be in charge. This seems to be true even in organizations made up of well-intentioned, idealistic members. Many of us, when placed in a position to do so, will fight for mastery over our fellows even as we speak earnestly in favor of equality. In OA, however, there are no powerful offices to hold. Instead of a power structure, we have a service structure. The offices or boards found in OA exist only to do service. They have no power to enforce rules on OA groups or individual members. In OA groups, members are chosen to perform services, such as keeping track of and distributing the group's money, finding speakers, attending intergroup or service board meetings, or restocking the literature table.

OA groups normally spend very little meeting time with group business. If somebody wants to make a change in the way a group is operating—to find a new meeting place, for instance, or to use some of the group's funds in a new way—this is brought up for discussion at a group conscience meeting of the group's regularly attending members. Some groups hold such meetings in conjunction with the regular meeting and some hold them separately. The informed group conscience decides what action is to be taken and individuals act for the group to implement this decision.

The group conscience is not the same as majority rule. This conscience is an expression of the group unity spoken of in the First Tradition, a common bond that grows among us as we each let go of self-will. Rather than being guided by individual self-interest, we seek as a group to apply the Principles embodied in OA's Steps, Traditions, and Concepts of Service to the decision at hand.

In order to reach an *informed* group conscience, we affirm each group member's right to take part in the discussions, and we listen to everyone attentively with open minds. The purpose of our discussions is to make sure that the decision reached by the group takes into account all pertinent information. If we are to reach an informed decision, the group needs to take into account everybody's ideas. For this reason, OA groups give all viewpoints a full hearing—even minority viewpoints.

All those who considers themselves a group member are welcome to speak or vote. Since, according to the Third OA Tradition,

"The only requirement for OA membership is a desire to st⟨ compulsively," OA groups do not place abstinence or other requ⟨⟩ ments on voting rights. How can we trust our group decisions if we allow people to vote who are eating compulsively and might not be clearheaded? This could certainly happen, but we need to keep OA open to all who want what our Fellowship has to offer. To exclude some from speaking or voting on decisions for the group denies them effective membership in the group, membership that can be essential to recovery from our "disease of isolation."

Those who have long-term experience with OA groups, Traditions, and Concepts have more than a right to speak up; they have a responsibility to share what they have learned. Sometimes they may hesitate for fear of being unpopular, but this information needs to be made known to all of us if we are to act wisely under the authority of a loving God.

Once all voices have been lovingly heard, a group conscience vote is taken. We each base our vote on what we believe is best for the group and OA as a whole, not on the personalities of those supporting a particular viewpoint, nor on what our closest friends believe.

In light of Tradition Two, nobody ever "loses" a group conscience vote in OA. Those of us whose opinions differed from the group decision may be disappointed and angry at first. Eventually, however, we often come to believe that the outcome was a good thing for us personally, as well as for OA. Whether we ever feel this way or not, the reality is that we all win when God's will is done.

Not all our group decisions will be wise and practical. We do make mistakes sometimes and have to look for better answers to a problem. Another group conscience vote can be taken when something needs to be corrected. Like individuals, OA groups learn from their mistakes—and so does OA as a whole. We find that our Higher Power often leads us through our blunders.

Members who have been around long enough to learn from such experiences are sometimes tempted to think their opinions should govern their groups, despite Tradition Two. When they try to control rather than to serve other members, however, things usually go wrong.

In starting a brand-new OA group, one or a few people might have to make all the decisions at first, but very soon the group conscience takes over the leadership function. The counsel of longtime members continues to be valuable, but it is not good for the group or its leaders if one person holds a particular service position too long. A vital part of our personal growth in OA is giving service, but it is also vital to practice humility by giving up our service office after a specified length of time so someone else can have this opportunity to carry the OA message.

Thus, service positions are rotated regularly in OA groups, even when the person holding the position has done a good job and would be willing to continue. This is somewhat disconcerting to the newcomer who may have taken it for granted that those performing services are in charge of the OA meeting. The first time a group secretary or program chair steps down from a position, a newcomer may feel as if the group is falling apart or being deserted by its leadership. After the newcomer returns to the meeting month after month, however, he or she begins to find security in the way the meeting is guided through its group conscience. Eventually, the member who regularly attends a meeting will decide to take part in group conscience discussions and decisions, find that the group continues to nurture his or her recovery despite changes, and see opportunities to give service. We take turns filling service offices in OA in the same way that family members might take turns doing household chores.[9]

All OA members share a responsibility for the operation of OA. Sometimes members who don't yet understand how our Fellowship works can be heard to say things like, "Why did they change my favorite pamphlet?" or "Why don't they have a meeting in my hometown?" We soon learn that there is no "they" and "them" in OA, only *we* and *us*. Acting through literature committees made up of OA

[9] The *OA Handbook for Members, Groups, and Service Bodies: Recovery Opportunities* (Overeaters Anonymous, Inc., © 1979 … 2015) offers many useful suggestions for OA groups and is available from the OA bookstore at bookstore.oa.org.

members from around the world, *we* decide what literature to publish and revise. If *we* want a meeting in town, it's up to those of *us* who want it there to start one. This kind of responsibility sometimes scares us, until we remember the words of Tradition Two. All we have to do is the footwork, and we can trust the outcome to our loving Higher Power who provides us with all the resources we need.

The first edition of *The Twelve Steps and Twelve Traditions of Overeaters Anonymous* is an example of how the Second Tradition works in OA. Before it was finished, approved by OA's World Service Business Conference, and published in its final form, the OA Fellowship went through a thirteen-year process in which we discussed—rather heatedly, at times—whether there was a need for the book and how it should be written. The text went through three major drafts and numerous revisions incorporating suggestions and comments from hundreds of OA members all over the world.

Several times during those years the entire project seemed doomed by controversy and confusion. Portions of the book were debated and voted on at World Service Business Conferences in 1987, 1989, 1990, 1992, and 1993 before the book was finally approved. During all those years, many of us wondered if a loving God as expressed in our group conscience could ever really get the book published. Each time, however, a series of events (often unexpected) would occur to solve the problems and get things back on track.

Many of us have had similar experiences in our home meetings. When a group problem is brought up for discussion, a better solution often arises from the workings of the group conscience than from any proposal the group's leaders are able to come up with on their own. As the discussion progresses, a whole new idea emerges, or from the back of the room, comes the voice of one of the newer members with a fresh idea for solving the problem. To our amazement, heated controversies, which threaten to split the group, are resolved, and we discover that the group has actually been strengthened in the process.

**How do we live up to the Principles of the Second Tradition in our OA meetings?**

*Does our group encourage everyone to take an active part in meetings and group conscience discussions?*

*Before voting on group conscience decisions, does the group take the time to find out as much as it can about the matter and discuss it fully? Do we listen with open minds to everyone's point of view?*

*Do we ever put pressure on the group to accept the ideas of certain individuals simply because they have been in OA a long time?*

*Do we feel like we have to control group discussions, or can we all go along in good spirit with the group conscience, even if we differed with it in the beginning?*

*Do we support our service officers, OA committees, and office workers, or do we sometimes criticize their efforts?*

*Do we hold our service officers accountable?*

*Does the group give full attention to the group secretary, intergroup or service board representative, and others making announcements?*

*Do our group's members volunteer or willingly accept group offices (e.g. secretary, treasurer), or does our group have trouble finding members willing to do service?*

*Do we all offer to help set up, clean up, or do other tasks, whether we are relatively new in OA or have been around a long time?*

Many of us come to OA with years of experience in trying to control our families, friendships, or work relationships by power or manipulation. We have been amazed by how well the Second Tradition works in OA, by what happens when we become willing simply to serve the group and let our Higher Power govern through the group conscience.

We find that most people are willing to cooperate cheerfully with decisions they help to make. Instead of arguing, sulking, nagging, or commanding, we learn in OA to state our needs and desires in an adult way and to let others tell us theirs, expressing our willingness to go along with any decision that takes everyone's needs into account. Anger and bitterness are often replaced by harmony and peace when we treat each person with respect and really listen to what everyone has to say. When this happens, a loving God's will is expressing itself through us and through our OA groups.

# TRADITION THREE

The only requirement for OA membership is a
desire to stop eating compulsively.

*SPIRITUAL PRINCIPLE*

### IDENTITY

Most organizations have a list of qualifications for membership, but in Overeaters Anonymous we have only one requirement: a desire to stop eating compulsively.

No person who has this desire can be barred from any OA group. OA members come from many different backgrounds, races, and religions. We can, and do, have differences in opinions, political views, values, lifestyles, age, gender, sexual orientation, and economic status. A person can never be too overweight, too underweight, or too normal in weight to be an OA member. Newcomers sometimes ask, "What if I only have ten pounds to lose?" The answer is there are no weight requirements of any kind in OA.

Nor is it a membership requirement to have common experiences with the disease of compulsive eating. Some of us tried many diets, while others of us never dieted at all. Some of us binged, and some didn't. Some of us fasted. Some of us purged by various methods. We count among our members those who have been eating compulsively since childhood and those who never had a problem with food until their retirement years. All who have experienced the pain of compulsive eating and want to stop are equally welcome here.

In OA, we even find a wide range of opinions about the program itself—about the Twelve Steps, the Twelve Traditions, and how best to apply them. Nobody is expelled from OA for not working the Steps, not getting a sponsor, not respecting the Traditions, or not adopting the Tools and practices many of us employ.

Does this mean the Steps, Traditions, Concepts, and Tools are unimportant? No, they are the vital difference between OA and all the other ways we have tried to deal with our compulsive eating. Recovery is a journey, and the Twelve Step program is the road we travel together in OA. The purpose of Tradition Three is to ensure that the road will always be accessible to all who wish to travel it. Thus, we say that any two or more compulsive eaters who come together to practice the Twelve Steps, and Twelve Traditions of OA, guided by the Twelve Concepts of OA Service, are considered an OA group, as long as they, as a group, have no other affiliations, do not require anyone to practice any actions to be a member, and register with the World Service Office.[10]

As Tradition Three implies, a desire to abstain—to refrain from compulsive eating and compulsive food behaviors—is at the heart of OA membership. There are many opinions among us about what it means, exactly, to stop eating compulsively. Nobody is excluded from OA membership because of her or his personal opinion of how to achieve abstinence. Note, too, that while the *desire* to stop eating compulsively is required, a person doesn't have to be abstinent to be welcome at OA meetings. We encourage one another to keep coming back, no matter what. In fact, many of us have kept coming back

---

[10] Refer to OA Inc., Bylaws Subpart B, Article V, Sections 1 and 2 for the full definition of a group.

to OA despite problems with abstinence and have found this to be the key to our recovery. In OA, the door never closes to a member who has returned to active compulsive eating, and many members who have maintained long-term abstinence had, at some time in the past, felt themselves to be hopeless because they had trouble staying abstinent or experienced a relapse.

Occasionally groups are plagued by members who disrupt the harmony of meetings. Of course groups must protect their members from violence or harassment. Groups have been known to confront a person acting in an abusive manner and ask her or him to leave the meeting. Even these people are not permanently barred from the group and denied the chance to recover.

Luckily, such extreme cases are rare. We have found that most personality problems can best be dealt with on a one-to-one basis. Our OA meetings aren't always going to be perfect, but we can find recovery in them despite their imperfections. When every person is respected and treated lovingly, the group survives and emerges stronger than ever from the experience.

Over the years, many OA groups have had participation requirements other than the simple desire to stop eating compulsively. In some, for instance, a person had to follow a certain food plan for a certain number of days in order to share in the meeting. In others, a person needed permission from a sponsor to share.

The question arose: Is this not a breach of the Third Tradition? If people must meet special requirements in order to have a voice in the meeting, aren't they being denied effective membership in the group? Generally, the group conscience of OA as a whole has agreed with this interpretation of Tradition Three, but there has been much discussion on this point. After all, the autonomy of groups is also a closely guarded OA Tradition, and groups having those kinds of requirements have been vital to the recovery of many of our members.[11]

In votes at the World Service Business Conferences in 1983, 1987, and 1989, delegates sought to formulate a way of dealing with

---

[11] See Tradition Four for how "group autonomy" relates to "other groups or OA as a whole."

this issue that would protect the autonomy of meetings and, at the same time, make sure that all compulsive overeaters can feel welcome in our Fellowship. The policy statement reads: "Overeaters Anonymous respects the autonomy of each OA group. We do suggest, however, that any group which imposes a special purpose, task, or guideline should inform its members that this special purpose, task, or guideline does not represent OA as a whole. The only requirement for membership is the desire to stop eating compulsively. Anyone who says they are a member is a member. We of Overeaters Anonymous welcome all members with open arms."[12]

Additional support of Tradition Three is shown in the adopted "Unity with Diversity" Policy, which encourages and promotes acceptance and inclusivity. A key point is the reminder that any member be allowed to "share his or her experience, strength, and hope in meetings regardless of the individual approach or specific concept that member may follow."[13]

Another policy was adopted in 2000 to clarify that members' inclusion at a meeting should not be restricted by whether or not they use a specific food plan.[14]

Some special-requirement meetings still exist within the OA Fellowship. For example, Step studies at which membership is limited and where participants must commit to attend regularly and complete assignments. Such support can be a boon to the OA member who needs extra help to reinforce her or his program. However, because of their special requirements or restrictions, these groups may not register as OA meetings with the OA World Service Office.

There are also special-focus groups in OA, such as those for men, women, gays and lesbians, and anorexics and bulimics. In cases where these groups are registered, they cannot exclude any compulsive eater who wants to attend and share.

---

[12] Overeaters Anonymous, Inc. Business Conference Policy Manual, Continuing Effect Motions 1983. Amended 1989.

[13] Overeaters Anonymous, Inc. Business Conference Policy Manual, Continuing Effect Motions 1992a. Amended 2013.

[14] Overeaters Anonymous, Inc. Business Conference Policy Manual, Continuing Effect Motions 2000a. Amended 2005.

We don't want to exclude any of our fellow sufferers or create barriers to their recovery. Many of us come to OA feeling like the rest of the world misunderstands compulsive overeaters and our problems. For us, OA is the only place where we truly feel we belong.

## How do we live by the Principles that underlie OA's Third Tradition?

*Does our group encourage everyone to take part in discussions?*

*Do we welcome every type of compulsive eater, or are there some types we would rather not have in OA or in our OA group?*

*Do we focus our discussions on the things we, as compulsive eaters, have in common?*

*Do we let people's age, race, education, manner of dress, weight, religion (or lack of it), political beliefs, language, gender, sexual orientation, or other factors determine whether we will reach out to them?*

*Are we overly impressed by an OA member's celebrity, professional status, or experience with other Twelve Step programs? Or, does the group treat each member equally?*

*Do we make it a point to speak to newcomers, even when their appearances or attitudes are not inviting? Do we let them know they are welcome in OA?*

*Does the group continue to extend a welcome to all compulsive eaters, even those who have been critical of group practices in the past?*

Before OA, we may have placed special requirements on our friends, coworkers, or family members. "I will love you if … " often characterized our attitude toward them. Perhaps we demanded that others live up to our standards or we placed conditions on friendships: "If you disagree with me, you have betrayed me." In OA, we've learned that people can differ with us on important matters and still be loving, supportive friends.

When we apply OA's Tradition Three, we find the treasure of

friendship often where we least expect it, with people we once would have excluded from our lives. Such treasure is all around us, and all we have to do is open our hearts to receive it. OA is where we learn to open our hearts, because it is here that most of us first experience unconditional acceptance. "We have a home, if we want it" is how "Our Invitation to You" in the *Overeaters Anonymous* book expresses Tradition Three. "Welcome to Overeaters Anonymous. Welcome home!"[15]

---

[15] *Overeaters Anonymous,* 3rd ed. (Overeaters Anonymous, Inc., © 1980 … 2014) p. 5.

# TRADITION FOUR

Each group should be autonomous except in matters
affecting other groups or OA as a whole.

---

*SPIRITUAL PRINCIPLE*

## AUTONOMY

A saying in Overeaters Anonymous is, "There are no musts in this program." As individuals, we are responsible for ourselves and free to work (or not work) the Twelve Step program however we wish. The same principle holds true for OA groups. Tradition Four—the Tradition of autonomy—gives OA groups the right and responsibility to operate as they see fit, free from any outside influence. Autonomy means that OA groups can have no affiliations, other than with OA. It also means that no other group or service body—even within OA—can dictate group action. There is only one limit to group autonomy in Tradition Four: Groups should not do anything that will injure other OA groups or OA as a whole.

Tradition Four gives OA groups the freedom to do what works best for them. Each group chooses its own meeting place and time, format, and practices. Every OA group makes its own decisions—and mistakes—without interference from any governing body other than its own group conscience.

Because groups are autonomous, OA members who visit meetings away from home often encounter group practices that seem strange to them. "These people aren't doing it right," the visitor thinks. "I miss my home group!" Sooner or later, however, the visitor discovers a delightful truth. OA meetings around the globe are alike in one respect: Every OA group operates in an atmosphere that promotes recovery from compulsive overeating through the Twelve Steps and Twelve Traditions of Overeaters Anonymous.

One very strong reason all groups are alike in spirit is found in the second half of Tradition Four. Autonomy extends only to matters that don't affect other OA groups or OA as a whole. What kinds of matters are likely to affect the entire OA Fellowship?

One instance would be a group that doesn't use the Twelve Steps and Twelve Traditions of OA as the basis for its meetings. By calling itself "OA" but not offering OA Principles to its members, this group would be misleading compulsive eaters about the OA program and harming the Fellowship as a whole. The Fellowship's definition of an OA group affirms this point: Any two or more compulsive overeaters who come together to practice the Twelve Steps and Twelve Traditions are considered a group, as long as that group has no other affiliations, does not require anyone to practice any actions to be a member, and is registered with the World Service Office.[16]

Groups that ignore one or more of the Twelve Traditions bring discord to the Fellowship. For example, groups have allowed disagreements to take precedence over sharing recovery in meetings. Other groups have continually depended on a handful of members for leadership, instead of trusting God to guide them through an informed group conscience. Some groups have limited their membership or set requirements for sharing, ignoring the Third Tradition. Or, groups have accepted rent-free meeting space, photocopying, or

---

[16] Refer to OA Inc., Bylaws Subpart B, Article V, Sections 1 and 2 for the full definition of a group.

other services from people and institutions outside OA, despite our Seventh Tradition of being self-supporting. Groups have promoted non-OA-approved literature to their members or focused meeting discussions on topics not related to recovery from compulsive eating, forgetting our primary purpose as expressed in Tradition Five. Meeting time has been used to promote outside enterprises and issues, despite our Sixth and Tenth Traditions. Groups and individuals have broken members' anonymity, even though two of our Traditions deal with this important aspect of our Fellowship. In these and many other ways, groups sometimes fail to live by the Principles embodied in our Twelve Traditions.

However, failure to uphold an OA Tradition does not result in a group being summarily ejected from the Fellowship—we might not have any OA Fellowship at all if that were the case!

When a group does not honor the Traditions, it's usually because members aren't well informed about them, not because they choose to ignore them. When the Traditions are not upheld, the positive atmosphere of the group begins to change. Enthusiasm and recovery wanes, members may decide to go elsewhere, and the survival of the group may be threatened. Therefore, when the Traditions are not being honored, it is essential that OA members who know them speak up to help the group understand them. A healthy discussion of the Twelve Traditions usually follows, and most groups elect to operate within these time-tested guidelines.

In extreme cases, where a group is affecting OA as a whole because of its persistent refusal to operate by OA Principles, the group may be deregistered from OA meeting lists, which are published by OA service bodies and the World Service Office. However, the service body taking such an action should do so only after much soul-searching. It is far too easy to use the power of the majority against groups in the minority simply because they have chosen a different approach to working the program, and not because they are truly harming other groups or OA as a whole by their actions. It is also easy for emotions and personality conflicts to enter into a decision not to list a certain OA meeting. When this happens, the Tradition of autonomy is ignored and the unity of the Fellowship suffers.

In 1988, OA's Board of Trustees decided not to register with the World Service Office any OA group that places special requirements on its members. At the same time, the board decided to allow the registration of groups that places specific abstinence or other requirements on officers or lead speakers, since these restrictions are not requirements for *membership* in the group. Still, the question arose whether this was a break of Tradition Four, which clearly states, OA "groups should be autonomous." To make sure group autonomy would be respected, it was decided that each group should judge whether the group's guidelines for attendance, sharing, or voting were suggestions or requirements.

Autonomy also means that OA groups operate free of outside influences. A meeting held in a church, office building, hospital, school, or other gathering place must conform to building rules concerning smoking, noise, tidiness, rent, parking, and the like. But we do not let others influence the OA group by limiting members' rights to express themselves in meetings. Nor can membership be confined to members of the church, employees of the company, patients at the hospital, residents of the area, or otherwise, since OA groups are open to all who have a desire to stop eating compulsively. Certainly, outside organizations should not be allowed to interject their practices into OA meetings.

In OA's early days, a group hosted by a large church had this experience. Unfamiliar with the Principle of autonomy, the group began to incorporate the church's healing practices into its meetings. Membership quickly soared to almost three hundred. Members of the group, convinced they had been forever healed of compulsive overeating, forgot about working the Steps. Soon they found themselves back in the throes of the disease. In a few months, the group dwindled to a handful, and eventually it disbanded.

Our fledgling Fellowship learned a lot from this experience. We saw that OA autonomy is essential if we are to live by our Traditions and keep OA's Twelve Step recovery program intact.

As our Fellowship has matured, OA groups have found ways

to meet their needs and still operate within the Twelve Traditions. Special-focus and special-topic meetings are examples of this. In OA, there are many special-focus meetings, such as Gay/Lesbian/Bi/ Trans, 100-Pounders, Anorexia/Bulimia, Young Persons, and more, which are composed of OA members who feel they can more readily identify with individuals with similar attributes. Special-topic meetings (*Lifeline,* Big Book, Literature Study, Maintenance, Meditation, etc.) have a defined topic of discussion. A list of both types of meetings is available by advanced search on the Find a Meeting page of oa.org. Groups have the autonomy to follow formats geared to their particular needs.

Group membership is open to all compulsive overeaters, however, and all members should be given an opportunity to share and have a say in how the meeting operates. Within these guidelines, special-focus and special-topic OA groups flourish and nurture the recovery of the individuals who belong to them.

The Fourth Tradition offers OA groups the freedom to find their own way and learn from their own experiences. At the same time, this Tradition assures all of us that our OA Fellowship won't be harmed by the misguided actions of one group and that OA meetings will continue to focus on the Principles embodied in OA's Twelve Steps and Twelve Traditions.

Living by the Fourth Tradition in OA means learning to act autonomously, even as we live in harmony with others. Here, we accept responsibility for ourselves, for our actions and their consequences, and for our own recovery. We learn to respect other OA members' autonomy when sponsoring or helping them. At the same time, we learn to accept other people's help without expecting them to do things for us that we should be doing for ourselves. We set necessary boundaries for ourselves and our OA groups so that we won't be abused by others, and we express our needs openly without insisting that others meet those needs in ways that might harm them.

**How well do we live by the Fourth Tradition?**

*Does our group feel there are only a few right ways of doing things in OA? Do we respect the right of other groups to have practices different from ours?*

*Does our group always consider the welfare of OA as a whole in making group conscience decisions? Do we do the same when voting how to spend our group's money, when planning OA group activities, or in the way we operate our meetings?*

*Do we stop to consider that our group's attitudes and actions may mold many newcomers' first impressions of OA as a whole?*

*Do we ever consider how our group's actions might affect the public's opinion about OA as a whole?*

*Does our group take time to discuss the Traditions? Do we take all Twelve Traditions into consideration when making group conscience decisions?*

*Do we keep our group free of control or influence from outside of OA?*

*Do we practice the Principle of autonomy by taking responsibility for our own actions and avoiding attempts to control the actions of others?*

All of us need the balance implicit in the Principle of autonomy to be the unique OA groups and individuals we are meant to be. Tradition Four challenges us as individuals, as OA groups, and as a Fellowship to strike a healthy balance between our responsibility for ourselves and our responsibility to each other, while we grow and work together as companions in recovery.

# TRADITION FIVE

Each group has but one primary purpose—
to carry its message to the compulsive overeater
who still suffers.

---

*SPIRITUAL PRINCIPLE*

**PURPOSE**

We compulsive overeaters have been offered a wide variety of solutions to our problems, from diet clubs and counseling programs to medications and surgeries. In the midst of all this competition for the overeater's attention and money, Overeaters Anonymous offers a spiritual program that has brought recovery to thousands who had lost hope. We who have found a sane way of eating and living have a responsibility to make sure OA doesn't become sidetracked. Our groups come together so we can share recovery through the Twelve Steps and the Twelve Traditions with fellow compulsive eaters. OA will always offer recovery to those suffering from our disease as long as we remember that this is our primary purpose.

One important reason we stick to our primary purpose in OA meetings is so our groups can help us practice the Twelfth Step. Experience has shown we cannot keep the precious gifts of our own recovery unless we give recovery away by sharing OA's message. When we focus our discussions on the Principles embodied in the Twelve Steps and Twelve Traditions, when we share how we've found the solution to our eating problems through practicing these Principles, we discover that we carry the message to those who still suffer, and to ourselves as well. No matter how much recovery we have, we still need to hear the OA message. Every time we offer our experience, strength, and hope to the still-suffering compulsive eater, we give back what we have been given and thus continue the flow of healing power that fosters our own recovery.

Further, we OA members have the ability to help our fellow compulsive overeaters in ways that no normal eater can. We know this because we have received so much valuable help from other OA members. Our doctors, families, or friends may have voiced their concerns about our eating problems or given us advice, but their words didn't help. We felt they didn't understand us. In OA, however, we found people who had done and felt the same things we had. We began to listen eagerly to what they had to say. We wanted to know how they were getting well. From these experiences, we discovered a key principle: The practicing compulsive overeater is more likely to find help from someone who has also experienced the pain of compulsive eating than from anyone else. Speaking openly about our own struggles from the perspective of our OA recovery, we bring the suffering newcomer the message of strength and hope that we have found in the OA Fellowship.

Tradition Five reminds us that our recovery doesn't come from simply discussing our problems with each other. It is in the OA message—in our Steps and Traditions—that we find solutions to our problems. Living by these Principles has saved our lives. *Honesty, hope, faith, courage, integrity, willingness, humility, self-discipline, love, perseverance, spiritual awareness, service, unity, trust, identity, autonomy, purpose, solidarity, responsibility, fellowship, structure, neutrality, anonymity,* and *spirituality:* These Principles, rather than our problems, should be the focus of every OA meeting. The same thing applies when we sponsor other OA members. We help them most when we listen, avoid giving advice, and share our experience with living by OA Principles.

An OA group is not a social club, though we make wonderful friends in OA and look forward to seeing them at meetings. Tradition Five reminds us that OA groups need to focus on meeting the needs of newcomers and struggling members. This includes personally welcoming them and explaining the basics of the OA recovery program. One OA member wrote in *Lifeline* of her experience with Tradition Five:

"In my first years in OA, meeting leaders would suggest that we introduce ourselves to newcomers at break time. Despite their numerous reminders, I never did, nor did many other members. God only knows how many newcomers walked out of those OA doors, never to return. We must have appeared quite cliquish to them.

"Things changed when my husband and I moved to a town where there were no OA meetings. My sponsor encouraged me to start one. I was scared, but I accepted the challenge. The group was small—only four of us—but we were eager to grow. We hoped for newcomers, but there weren't any.

"Soon we learned that two of our four members would have to drop out because of scheduling conflicts. But before they left, we got our first newcomer! We fell all over her. At the break, *everybody* went up to talk to her. Suddenly I found that my fear of approaching a new person had vanished. My need for recovery far outweighed my fear.

"These days I no longer avoid talking to newcomers. I now approach them with open arms, thank them for coming, and encourage them to return. Without them, this group of ours wouldn't be celebrating its first anniversary!"[17]

---

[17] "Vital Connection," *Lifeline,* © March 1990, pp. 20–21.

The "compulsive overeater who still suffers" isn't always a new-comer to OA. She or he can also be an established member experiencing difficulties with the disease of compulsive eating or with other problems. Seeing one of our members go into relapse or face personal problems can be frightening to us. We may instinctively react by not reaching out or avoiding them at meetings.

When we act in these ways, we're forgetting the primary purpose of our group, which is to carry OA's message of hope to those who still suffer—including those among us who have heard the message many times before.

Tradition Five also tells us to look beyond our own group, to compulsive overeaters who have not yet attended a meeting. Our primary purpose includes a responsibility to reach out to these people in whatever ways we can. This is the reason each OA group spends a part of its funds supporting intergroups, service boards, regions, and world services. Service bodies and world services extend the hand and heart of OA into the world around us in ways that individual groups often cannot: by maintaining websites and answering services, by placing meeting notices and information about OA in the media, by staging special events, by publishing meeting lists and literature, by providing speakers and information for healthcare, professional, and public events, and in many other ways.

Before OA many of us simply lived to eat. Now that we've joined together in OA groups, we have a new purpose.

---

**How are we making decisions that help us carry a message of hope and recovery to others?**

*Does our group concentrate sufficiently on OA's primary purpose? Do we focus our discussions on the Twelve Steps, the Twelve Traditions, the Tools, and recovery from compulsive eating? Or do we just talk about the events of our lives without sharing how the program is helping us to change?*

*Do we welcome newcomers to our group and give them individual attention?*

*Do we try to make the OA Fellowship known to people outside who need help? In what ways do we support our intergroup, service board, region, and world services in our efforts to reach out?*

*Do we ever volunteer to help newcomers, visitors, or other members who need transportation to attend our meetings?*

*What do we do to welcome back members who are returning to OA?*

*Do we make a point to welcome new members, talk with them, and offer phone numbers?*

*Can members find sponsors in our group?*

*Does anybody in our group make a point to call newcomers or members who have been missing from the meeting?*

*Do we remember longtime OA members who still suffer physically, emotionally, or spiritually? How do we treat the member who is facing difficulties with compulsive eating or with life?*

For OA groups and members alike, the Fifth Tradition helps us to keep it simple. We find that when we focus on our primary objective of carrying the message of recovery, we are empowered to use our talents in ways that are truly useful to others. The result is better than any outcome we could have planned for ourselves, for we find a deep satisfaction in service as we join forces to share recovery in OA.

# TRADITION SIX

An OA group ought never endorse, finance,
or lend the OA name to any related facility or outside
enterprise, lest problems of money, property,
and prestige divert us from our primary purpose.

---

*SPIRITUAL PRINCIPLE*

## SOLIDARITY

Tradition Five defines our primary purpose. Tradition Six cautions each OA group to stick to the primary purpose exclusively, no matter how many outside enterprises may interest us as individuals.

Our Fellowship has been invited to affiliate with many outside enterprises, from treatment centers and health spas to cookbooks. Misguided OA members have been known to use our telephone lists to solicit sales. Members who are unfamiliar with Traditions Five and Six sometimes promote outside enterprises in OA meetings—everything from books and vitamins to treatment programs and church revivals.

Many of these enterprises may be helpful and deserving of attention and support. Why, then, do OA groups make it a practice to say no to all such outside endeavors? The reason can be summarized in three words: *Keep it simple.* Though these enterprises may be worthwhile, they threaten to divert the attention of groups from OA's primary purpose, which is to carry the message of Twelve Step recovery to compulsive overeaters who still suffer.

Before OA had its own literature, some groups gave away or sold a variety of non-OA-approved material. Since OA now publishes its own literature, the group conscience of OA suggests that all groups use, sell, and display only OA-approved literature at meetings and OA-sponsored events.[18] Whenever an OA meeting uses, sells, or displays non-OA-approved literature, it implies that OA endorses the philosophy of that author. OA-approved literature reflects the experience of many members of the Fellowship whose recovery is strongly rooted in the Twelve Steps and Twelve Traditions.

The Sixth Tradition helps OA groups fulfill our primary purpose of carrying the OA message. If meeting time is taken up by the promotion of outside enterprises or other Twelve Step programs, if newcomers can't tell the outside literature from the OA literature at our meetings, if members put their phone numbers on OA phone lists only to be bothered by sales calls, the OA message of recovery soon gets lost. Those who suffer from the misery of compulsive eating need to hear about the solution found in working the Twelve Steps during our meetings and phone calls. They also need to know that there are no strings attached, no gimmicks, no stockholders demanding that money be made.

There are many treatment programs for people with eating disorders available outside OA. Many recognize the value of the Twelve Steps and take measures to involve their clients or patients in OA meetings. Although outside enterprises may endorse OA, OA does not endorse any of those outside enterprises. We welcome all who

---

[18] Statement on Approved Literature, Overeaters Anonymous, Inc. Business Conference Policy Manual, Continuing Effect Motions 2010a. Amended 2012.

come to our meetings with a desire to stop eating compulsively, no matter what other forms of treatment they might be involved in as individuals. OA has no affiliation with any form of treatment or therapy.

OA groups often meet in facilities belonging to an outside enterprise, such as a church, hospital, government agency, or company. This implies no affiliation with the entity that owns the building where the group meets. OA groups pay rent for the use of meeting space in buildings owned by outside enterprises.

In one city, a hospital opened an eating disorders unit, began bringing its patients to OA meetings on a regular basis, and then convinced one OA group to move its meeting place into the hospital's conference room. Many former patients of the unit soon became staunch OA members, and often speakers at the OA meetings would mention the hospital program by name when sharing their stories. Soon, speakers, some not long out of treatment and not yet familiar with the Traditions, were promoting the hospital program in the OA meeting. This began to happen so frequently that newcomers were given the impression OA endorsed this other program. At this point, an OA veteran objected, pointing out OA's Sixth Tradition of not endorsing outside enterprises. A heated group conscience discussion took place.

"How can you be so ungrateful to the hospital after all the support they've given OA?" asked one member. "Besides, my treatment there brought me to OA. I'm sharing my personal experience."

The matter was resolved happily with a simple suggestion. OA members need to be free to share their experience, but the group now asks its speakers to refrain from stressing the names of any specific outside enterprises, including the hospital's eating disorders treatment program.

In addition to treatment programs, there are bookstores full of recovery literature for compulsive eaters, Twelve Step ministries, counselors, retreats, and therapy groups. One crucial difference between these and OA groups is that, while many of them are based on the Twelve Steps, they don't govern themselves according to the

Twelve Traditions. For instance, they may have professionals in positions of authority, they may have requirements for participation beyond a desire to stop eating compulsively, or they may have the profit motive as a primary purpose.

Many of these programs have been helpful to OA members, and we're grateful that as individuals we have so many choices to assist us in our recovery and spiritual growth. Certainly, we are free to supplement our personal recovery in OA with other kinds of support. Still, following Tradition Six, OA groups do not affiliate with any non-OA enterprises. We take whatever measures we can to make sure they don't use the OA name, and we avoid using OA meeting time and space to promote them.

Nor is OA affiliated with other Twelve Step and Twelve Tradition fellowships, although many of us are also members of them. OA has sometimes made use of the wisdom and experience of other Twelve Step groups in making decisions for our Fellowship, but we are not a part of any of them, nor they of us. We have our own purpose to fulfill—providing a Twelve Step and Twelve Tradition Fellowship for compulsive overeaters.

As discussed in relation to Tradition Five, OA meetings focus on recovery from compulsive overeating. Members who put too much emphasis on other fellowships in OA meetings leave compulsive eaters with the impression that these programs and the problems they address are more serious or more important to the compulsive eater than OA. Such is not the case, and keeping the Sixth Tradition means that we refrain from promoting other programs in OA meetings.

OA's lack of attachment to any kind of outside enterprise gives our Fellowship a marvelous freedom. We operate with a minimum of worry about funding, administrative problems, or the success and failure of non-OA ventures. By avoiding any such affiliations, OA groups can concentrate on recovery from compulsive eating instead of on problems associated with money, property, and prestige, which cause so much conflict in the world around us.

### How do we respect OA's Sixth Tradition?

*Does our group discourage members from promoting outside enterprises in OA meetings? Or do we rationalize that people need to hear about the outside program being discussed, so it won't hurt if we ignore the Traditions this time?*

*When we vote on how to use group funds and other resources, are we careful to avoid financing outside enterprises?*

*Does our group use, sell, or display outside literature at our meetings?*

*Are we careful never to use our OA group contacts for personal financial gain? Do we speak up when we see somebody else misusing OA phone lists and/or meetings in such a way?*

*When we share in meetings, are we careful not to imply an OA endorsement of outside enterprises, such as hospitals, eating disorders treatment programs, other Twelve Step fellowships, books, publications, and other resources?*

When we find ourselves or our OA groups embroiled in problems of money, property, and prestige, we have a clue that we might have involved ourselves in matters that would be better left alone. We cause these kinds of problems when we take on outside responsibilities or promote outside causes, diverting our group's attention and resources from OA's primary purpose of carrying the OA message.

"First things first" is another slogan that sums up Tradition Six. In OA, we learn to focus on our primary purpose and exclude from our groups everything that might interfere with our ability to carry the OA message.

# TRADITION SEVEN

Every OA group ought to be fully self-supporting,
declining outside contributions.

---

*SPIRITUAL PRINCIPLE*

## RESPONSIBILITY

Tradition Seven follows naturally from Traditions Five and Six. If the Overeaters Anonymous Fellowship is to fulfill our primary purpose and remain free of outside influences, we must stay free of the need for outside contributions as well. Thus, OA ought to be fully self-supporting.

Money is needed to keep the OA program alive. Each group has expenses, such as rent and literature. When individual groups join to form an intergroup or service board, opportunities to carry the OA message multiply, but so do expenses. Intergroups and service boards may provide meeting lists, have phone lines or answering services, maintain websites, distribute information about the OA program in their communities, publish newsletters, and organize events.

OA regions stage events; publish newsletters; help new groups, intergroups, or service boards get established; and carry the message in many other ways throughout their area. In keeping with Tradition Eight, OA's World Service Office employs special workers. These employees provide services that play a vital part in each member's individual recovery. These include publishing OA books, pamphlets, and *Lifeline,* our magazine of recovery; maintaining the OA website and worldwide meeting lists; and answering inquiries from all over the world about our program.

All of these efforts are paid for by *us,* OA members who make contributions. Nobody is charged dues or fees at an OA meeting. We collect the "Seventh Tradition," and most of us are glad to contribute to keep our own groups and our Fellowship afloat. After all, OA is our life preserver, our means of recovery from the disease of compulsive eating.

Tradition Seven tells us that the financial support of OA is our responsibility as members of the Fellowship. We don't ask for or accept support from outside sources. There is also a limit on the amount that may be given by one member in one year to OA's World Service Office.

The reason for this is clear. If we accept "free" gifts from outsiders, or too much from one member, it threatens our autonomy. We may become dependent on these funds and never learn to take responsibility and pay our share. The need to maintain good relations with the donor could then divert attention from our primary purpose. Meanwhile, those who are paying OA's way might naturally expect to influence our decisions. And those giving large amounts might feel they have a right to dominate the group. In these situations, we need to remember that our ultimate authority is a loving God as expressed in our group conscience.

Money is necessary to keep all levels of OA service operating. In keeping with Tradition Seven, we pay all group expenses out of group funds, whether or not they be for rent, literature, or supplies. Excess funds inevitably cause problems at any service level, therefore when a group or service body has more than sufficient funds for their needs, they set aside a prudent reserve for short-term expenses and forward the surplus funds to support the financial needs of OA as a whole. The service bodies and World Service Office use this financial support to continue carrying the message in ways groups cannot.

In one case, a group had been meeting harmoniously and growing rapidly for a year, but had never made a contribution to its intergroup. Funds in the group treasury were well over the amount needed to pay the next few months' rent and the literature table was well stocked. Finally, the group's treasurer brought up the subject of the excess funds. "We need more fun in our lives," she said. "Let's take that money and throw a party!"

Other members objected. "Mark, our group secretary, is moving out of town," one said. "We should buy him a nice going-away present with that money." Soon the group was embroiled in a dispute about how the excess funds should be spent.

Finally, one member offered another thought. "I found out about this meeting when I called our intergroup's phone line. Shouldn't we be sending the excess funds to intergroup to help pay for the phone and other services?" After a discussion of Traditions Five and Seven, the group voted to keep enough of the money to cover expenses for the next three months and to send the remainder on to help the intergroup, region, and World Service Office carry OA's message.

Another group, seeking to avoid accumulating excess funds, went to the other extreme and simply stopped collecting contributions for a while. This solved the excess money problem but kept the group from making needed contributions to its service bodies or the World Service Office.

One week a member pointed this out to the group. But a second member objected. "The Seventh Tradition says to be *self*-supporting. It doesn't say anything about supporting service bodies or the World Service Office."

"Aren't those groups working for *us?*" a third member asked. "They tell newcomers what OA is and how to find our meeting. If we don't do our share to support them financially, how can we claim to be fully self-supporting?"

During the next week, members of the group thought about the conventions and events, publications and meeting lists, website information and maintenance, and other help, information, and support that had been provided to their group by OA service bodies. "Intergroup, region, and world services are parts of our group, too," they agreed. And they voted to start collecting money again so they could contribute their share of the funds needed to keep these service bodies and the World Service Office going.[19]

In cases where a group is struggling financially, the Fellowship as a whole might be glad to cover expenses for the fledgling meeting for a while. Over time, however, this kind of dependency becomes unhealthy. As soon as possible, OA groups need to pay their share of the costs for the services they receive from OA service bodies and the World Service Office. The same principle applies to individuals in OA. Even those of us experiencing financial struggles find we need to make some contribution to our OA meetings. For many of us, our willingness to pay our own way is a sign that we are recovering and maturing emotionally.

The Seventh Tradition doesn't apply simply to financial support, however. Intergroups or service boards are made up of representatives from the groups that come together to undertake activities that will carry OA's message of recovery to those who still suffer. To be fully self-supporting, groups and individuals need to take on their share of this important service work. Financial contributions may pay for a phone line or website, but somebody in OA needs to return the calls and maintain the site. Money may be needed to provide newsletters, but first, OA members have to write, edit, and design them. Groups need to send representatives to their intergroup or service board meetings to participate in the decision making, as well as to bring back information and materials to their meetings. Individuals must volunteer to help if the service body is to host conventions or other events. Our intergroups and service boards need

---

[19] See *Seventh Tradition of OA* (Overeaters Anonymous, Inc., © 2016) for information on how groups may distribute contributions to service bodies and the World Service Office.

chairs, secretaries, treasurers, region representatives, and World Service Business Conference delegates. Meetings are fully self-supporting only when they contribute their share of the work that goes into carrying OA's message areawide, regionwide, and worldwide. We, as individuals, are fully self-supporting only when we do what we can, when we can, giving back some of the help we have been given in OA.

Even as there is a limit to the amount of money any one member may contribute, there should also be healthy limits for giving service. When one member, or a small handful of members, continually does all the work, resentments usually arise. Other members may feel excluded, so that OA divides into two groups—the "insiders" and the "outsiders." The insiders feel overwhelmed with service work and underappreciated. The outsiders resent the insiders for trying to control everything.

One OA group was started by a member who continued to do all the service work in the group for more than two years. She kept the key and unlocked the door, led the meetings, recorded the funds, and represented the group at intergroup. She was puzzled, however, that her group never grew. In fact, it gradually dwindled until, finally, during the group's second summer, everybody except the founder quit coming. As she sat there by herself for the third week in a row, she examined her service work in light of what she knew about OA's Traditions. "I think my Higher Power is trying to tell me something," she said to the empty chairs in front of her. "Maybe I need to let go of control here and let God take over this meeting."

The following week, another member showed up early for the meeting and asked if she could have the key. "I need to do more service work," she said. "Having the key will ensure that I get to the meeting." The founder needed no further clues to her Higher Power's will. She got others to lead the meetings, and the group elected a new secretary, treasurer, and intergroup representative. Never again did she have to sit in the room by herself and wonder what had gone wrong with the group.

The principle of being fully self-supporting is an important one for OA groups and recovering compulsive eaters. In the OA group, we learn to depend on God for our security, rather than on other people. Under the guidance of our Higher Power, we learn to do the things we need to do to take care of ourselves and our groups, materially and emotionally. We begin to look to our Higher Power rather than to other people as the source of our happiness and security.

Paradoxically, being fully self-supporting means we are now free to ask for help in doing OA service and in other matters as well. In light of the Seventh Tradition, we begin to see more clearly what our boundaries need to be. We begin to share our vulnerability with others in OA without expecting them to shoulder our responsibilities. As our Higher Power helps us to be self-supporting, we can let go of our unhealthy dependencies and develop healthy relationships with the people who share our lives.

---

### How well do we practice OA's Seventh Tradition?

*Do we really contribute all we can to OA's financial support?*

*When contributing to the Seventh Tradition, do we remember how much we spent on each binge? How much money we spent on weight-loss attempts that didn't work?*

*Are those of us who are recovering financially willing to contribute a little more?*

*Do we contribute something to the group's funds, trusting in our Higher Power, even when we're afraid of economic insecurity?*

*Does our group consider the group treasurer's job an important one and take care to make sure it is being done in a responsible manner? Do we listen carefully to the treasurer's report?*

*Does our group pay its own expenses out of its funds? Do we pay the going rate for rent at our meeting place? Do we pay for copying our phone lists, or do we expect somebody's employer to donate that?*

*Does our group regularly contribute to our service bodies and the World Service Office to support carrying the OA message?*

Doing our share of the service work is also part of being fully self-supporting.

*Does our group send a representative to each intergroup or service board meeting?*

*Does our intergroup or service board send representatives to region assemblies and delegates to the World Service Business Conference?*

*As members of a virtual group using the services of the World Service Office, do we accept our responsibility to help support OA by contributing directly?*

*Do we expect every member of our group to take a turn at doing OA service work?*

*Do we rotate jobs regularly, or do we have the same people doing the same services year after year?*

*Do some members take on more OA service jobs than they can effectively handle at one time? Do we encourage less active members to become more involved?*

The Seventh Tradition of saying no to outside contributions and yes to our responsibilities as OA groups and individuals is a vital principle. It keeps us and our Fellowship free of the complications that would inevitably arise were we to depend on outside sources, and when we honor this Tradition, we gain the self-respect that comes from being fully self-supporting.

# TRADITION EIGHT

Overeaters Anonymous should remain forever nonprofessional, but our service centers may employ special workers.

---

*SPIRITUAL PRINCIPLE*

**FELLOWSHIP**

Overeaters Anonymous is built on a foundation of sharing our experience, strength, and hope, one member to another. As OA members, we may serve each other by sponsoring, speaking at meetings, and doing necessary committee and other service work. For this, none of us receive payment in money. Our reward is something money can't buy—our own personal recovery.

The tradition of nonprofessionalism helps OA steer clear of the profit motive and concentrate on offering Twelve Step recovery to all who seek it. Newcomers to OA are often impressed by the honesty they hear, the depth of sharing, and the spirit of compassion found at OA meetings. None of us are paid to be here. Each of us is a compulsive eater, and we all come seeking support for our own personal recovery. Knowing this, we can trust each other to speak from the heart, to share what our experience has taught us, and to listen compassionately to our fellow members.

Since there are no professional OA members, we all have an equal opportunity to serve our fellow compulsive eater. We don't need certification, education, or credentials to share our program or to do service. All we need is willingness and a commitment to the Twelve Steps and Twelve Traditions of OA. Each of us can play a key role. Since our Twelfth Step includes carrying the OA message, it's good that there are plenty of opportunities for all of us to be of service.

When services demand special skills, professionals are hired for their expertise or advice. Tradition Eight says, "our service centers may employ special workers." Our experience has shown that some paid employees are necessary to take care of the business of OA.

For instance, in one city the intergroup decided to open an office. A nonprofessional volunteer was found to manage the office, making sure correspondence was attended to, bills were paid, the phone was answered, supplies were ordered, and records were maintained. After several months of faithful service, the volunteer manager got sick and had to resign. The intergroup began looking for a new volunteer. Two months went by, and the position was not filled. "I'd like to help out," people would say, "but I just don't have time to do that much service." Finally, five OA members agreed to take care of parts of the task, staffing the office in shifts. This arrangement was better than no office management at all, but the office was still in a state of confusion. Details were continually overlooked, and volunteers often had to put aside the office's business to take care of other priorities in their lives. Nobody, not even the landlord, knew who was in charge or whom to call when a problem arose. At last, the intergroup accepted the fact that the office manager's job was too big to be handled by volunteers and too important to be left to chance.

"We can't afford it," they said, "but we're going to have to hire a manager."

So hire a manager they did. Although it wasn't a requirement that the manager be an OA member, they decided to look first among their membership, since a manager who was also in OA would need less training in order to answer inquiries about the Fellowship. A recovering member with the necessary business skills was found to manage the office for a reasonable salary, and in that city, OA had its first-ever paid employee. Effective office management helped OA grow stronger there, and the growing membership was glad to pay the manager for a job well done.

However, we are never paid for the service we give in OA—the hours we spend carrying the message of recovery to other compulsive overeaters. Members who lead OA-sponsored retreats or events are reimbursed for their travel and lodging expenses but are not paid for their leadership, even if they are professionals who command a fee in non-OA settings.

Some OA members have worked for hospitals and eating disorders treatment centers as professional therapists and have found their OA experience to be of great value to them in this work. The question arises whether they are breaking the Eighth Tradition by accepting pay for working with eating disorder sufferers. Such people, however, are being paid for their work as professional therapists, not as professional OA members. To be sure, they may speak with their clients about their OA experience. But in the therapy groups they conduct professionally, they are in authority. They are responsible for applying their expertise in the field of psychology to the needs of their clients. When they attend OA meetings, they are simply OA members with no greater authority than any other member of the group, and they are free to focus on their own recovery. At OA functions, they are requested to speak only about their personal recovery to avoid implying endorsement of an outside enterprise by OA as a whole.

OA meetings are often very therapeutic, but they are not the same as therapy groups. One major difference between OA groups and therapy groups can be seen in the Eighth Tradition. OA has no professional therapists charged with responsibility for guiding and working with members of the group. Though most of us feel free to share our problems at OA meetings, providing psychotherapy is not the purpose of OA. During the recovery process, some of us have found we needed the help of a therapy group with professional leadership, in addition to OA. By working through some of our problems in therapy, we've been able to get our specific needs met while we continue to focus on the Twelve Steps in our OA meetings.

The vast good OA does for suffering compulsive eaters worldwide is still, for the most part, done nonprofessionally by OA members who give back what they are so generously given. This spirit of caring and sharing is one of the greatest strengths we have to offer as a Fellowship, for it carries with it a true healing power.

In OA, we learn to give our loving support to others freely, without trying to advise people or change them; nor do we look to others to work our program for us. In keeping with our nonprofessional status in OA, we willingly share and listen to our fellow compulsive eaters, but we try to leave behind expectations that they should solve our problems for us, that we should solve theirs, or that others will repay us in some way for helping them. Service is its own reward. When we approach others in this way, we often find that they respond to us with a new depth of love and trust.

---

**How well are we learning to live by the principle of nonprofessionalism in OA?**

*Do we sometimes try to "fix" other people in OA meetings by giving them our "expert advice," or are we content to share our own experience, strength, and hope?*

*Do we try to speak as experts in OA meetings or when sponsoring? On recovery? On health issues and medicine? Or on nutrition? On the Big Book? On the OA Fellowship or program? On psychology? On spiritual matters? Or, even on humility?*

*When we're having trouble with the program, do we try to hide that from those we sponsor or from our OA group because of our pride, shame, or fear?*

*Do we consider other OA members to be experts or authorities because of their experience, reputation, or personal magnetism?*

*Do we ever treat some of our members as professionals, forgetting that they come to OA for their own recovery?*

*Do we make other people responsible for our abstinence or other aspects of our recovery?*

*Can we distinguish what OA employees do from what members do in sharing their personal experience, strength, and hope?*

*Can we distinguish what therapists and workers in eating disorders treatment programs do from OA sharing?*

When we keep OA's Eighth Tradition, we discover a beautiful spirit of caring service, which becomes a powerful factor in our healing. We are all nonprofessionals in our support of each other's recovery from compulsive eating, giving and receiving support and fellowship with no expectations of return. Living by the spirit of this Tradition, we can each turn to the one next to us and say truthfully from the heart, "I put my hand in yours because I care."

# TRADITION NINE

OA, as such, ought never be organized;
but we may create service boards or committees
directly responsible to those they serve.

---

*SPIRITUAL PRINCIPLE*

## STRUCTURE

Visitors to Overeaters Anonymous meetings sometimes shake their heads and say, "Tradition Nine is the Tradition these people adhere to the closest. This group is never organized!"

Though our OA meetings may seem chaotic at times, chaos isn't the goal of Tradition Nine. What this Tradition encourages us to do is remain as free as possible from the bureaucracy that tends to form around organizations. In such instances, the organization and administration takes on a life of its own and obscures the real purpose of the group. Everything we do in OA is geared to our primary purpose of carrying our message of recovery based on spiritual Principles. Taking care of group business is very important. Still, as little meeting time as possible is spent electing service officers, voting on issues, organizing events, or making reports. Instead, we concentrate on sharing our experience, strength, and hope with each other and on studying the Steps and Traditions.

In order to keep our meeting time as free as possible from organizational activities, OA groups create service bodies, such as intergroups and service boards. When a group affiliates with an intergroup or a service board, it gives the group a voice in OA as a whole. These intergroups and service boards conduct business, such as coordinating local public information activities, maintaining websites, publishing newsletters, and planning special events. They have elected officers and bylaws by which they operate. OA groups that have joined to form an intergroup or a service board send a representative to the meetings to participate in business decisions, get feedback on group issues, and report back to their groups what the intergroup or service board is doing.

Though our service bodies need to be organized, OA is encouraged by Tradition Nine to keep the emphasis on fellowship, rather than organization. This Tradition helps to ensure that God always remains our ultimate authority in OA. Without an organized power structure in which to operate, no single person or group of people can govern others. No rules can be laid down, no punishments handed out, no orders issued. To be sure, service bodies and the World Service Office can drop from their meeting lists groups that continuously ignore our Traditions, but no OA group can be fined or ordered to disband. OA groups don't operate under any charter from the World Service Office or anyone else. On the contrary, world services derives its authority from the thousands of OA groups all over the world.

Nor can any individual member be kicked out of OA. Members come and go at will, contributing as much or as little as they see fit, and no power structure exists to require otherwise. Our experience has shown that unless we live by the spiritual Principles embodied in the Steps, Traditions, and Concepts of OA Service, no amount of organization will prevent chaos in OA. Our personal and group survival depends on adherence to these Principles, not on obedience to any power structure.

This Tradition of "nonorganization" can be very disconcerting to those of us who long for perfect meetings that always operate smoothly according to rules everybody understands. Some of us feel insecure when we discover there are no rules, only suggestions and Traditions, and no leaders with authority to enforce these Traditions. After we've been around for a while, however, we begin to see that this kind of human-powered organization isn't necessary after all. Meetings that are far from perfect in our eyes can still offer us the miracle of recovery. Our groups make mistakes, but most manage to survive. In fact, we find we can learn from these mistakes and grow stronger.

After observing this Tradition in operation for a while, most of us begin to trust that there really is a Higher Power guiding the OA Fellowship through our group conscience. We can relax, trust God, and appreciate the wisdom of the Ninth Tradition.

Does this mean we say nothing when our groups disregard the Traditions? Quite the opposite! When Traditions are not honored, individuals have a responsibility to speak up—lovingly and clearly—even when we may make ourselves unpopular with other members of the group by doing so. When members ignore the Traditions, it is often because they don't understand them or the spiritual Principles on which the Traditions are based. By speaking when a Tradition is not honored, we help other OA members learn about these spiritual Principles. It's one very important way we share our experience in OA.

Once we've spoken, however, we need to accept that conflict may result, that our words might not be heeded, and that we have no way of enforcing our understanding of the Traditions within the group. We speak in favor of the Traditions as best we can, leaving the results to our Higher Power.

One member wrote in *Lifeline* about how she spoke up for the Traditions in a meeting: "Our leader for the meeting wanted to read to us from a little booklet by a religious leader. Before she began, she said, 'I know this isn't OA-approved literature, but does anyone object to my reading it to the group?'

"I quietly responded, 'You *know* I'm going to object. Our primary purpose during an OA meeting is to carry the OA message. We can do as we like outside of meetings.'

"With that, the other members in the room urged her to do as she wished, as she was the leader. A newcomer wondered why we shouldn't be allowed to share anything we thought might help. Several people were irritated by my objection and a comment was made about the need to be open-minded.

"The reading was awkwardly deleted and we proceeded with a less than serene meeting. Afterwards I was told that I'd made others feel it was too risky to volunteer to lead.

"As I experience the isolation and pain of standing up for my convictions, I am filled with questions: 'Was I being a trusted servant, willing to speak up for the Traditions? If we resort to doing whatever we want to in a meeting, is it an Overeaters Anonymous meeting, or an Anything-Goes Anonymous meeting?' "[20]

Most veteran OA members have found that standing up for our Traditions is worth the risk that we'll be criticized or that meetings might be "less than serene." The alternative could be something worse for us than temporary unpopularity and conflict. It could be that, if we were to sit by and say nothing while our Traditions were ignored, OA meetings would lose their focus on the Principles of the Twelve Step program. The great healing power we have found in these meeting rooms would no longer be here for us. Living by OA's Ninth Tradition means that we don't depend on some authority or power structure to enforce the Traditions. We all take responsibility to speak when they are being ignored.

In the same way, the Ninth Tradition doesn't mean that OA groups should never make guidelines for conduct at their meetings. When problems arise—problems having to do with such issues as meeting format, smoking, cross talk—groups often hold group

---

[20] "Since You Asked..." *Lifeline,* © November 1990, p. 19.

conscience meetings to find solutions. Some groups hold these meetings apart from regular meeting time, so that they won't take up minutes needed for sharing; other groups hold group conscience discussions and votes during the regular meeting, so all the group's members are able to take part. Individuals who have a healthy respect for the group conscience follow the guidelines the group has decided on. As with our Traditions, when individuals ignore the group conscience, every member has the right and responsibility to speak up.

Once we have spoken our minds, however, the Ninth Tradition guides us to relax and let our Higher Power take charge of the meeting. We find we cannot force our will on the OA group, no matter how right it may seem to us.

### How well do we practice Tradition Nine?

*Does our group support those who do service or are we critical of them and suspicious of their motives?*

*Are we mature enough to take personal responsibility for the well-being of OA and for our own recovery? Or, do we expect "them" to take care of things for us?*

*Do we try to understand and support OA's service structure? Do we do our part in helping OA's service bodies and world services to carry the message?*

*Do we use patience and humility in performing each OA job we take?*

*Are we aware of all those to whom we are responsible when serving in any OA job?*

*Has our group made it a point to discuss the Twelve Traditions and how they apply to us?*

*Are we afraid to speak up when we see Traditions being ignored in our OA group or service body?*

*When doing OA service, can we trust the results to our Higher Power, even when things don't go the way we think they should?*

*Do we practice rotation of service in our groups and service bodies? Do we discuss how rotation of service relates to personal humility and the OA Principle of anonymity?*

In Overeaters Anonymous, we have experienced how things work out for the best when organization is kept at a minimum. The order we once sought in rules and power structures, we have found in freedom instead. Trusting our Higher Power rather than any organizational structure, we can now take responsibility for our shared lives and for the OA Fellowship in which we are recovering together.

# TRADITION TEN

Overeaters Anonymous has no opinion on outside issues; hence the OA name ought never be drawn into public controversy.

---

*SPIRITUAL PRINCIPLE*

## NEUTRALITY

We live in a world that thrives on controversy. When we arrive at OA and first hear OA's Tenth Tradition, it comes as a surprise to many of us that this organization, so supportive of our recovery from compulsive eating, will not be moved to throw its moral weight behind other good causes. How can OA sit by and say nothing about the many social evils that seem to go unchecked in our world?

The reason is simple. Our members come from many areas and backgrounds, and we have many shades of opinion on every issue. If OA were to take a stand on any one of these, we could immediately alienate some of our own membership as well as many of our fellow sufferers outside of OA. By allowing controversy over outside issues to drive away people who need the recovery OA has to offer, we would take a step backward from our primary objective of carrying our message to the compulsive overeater who still suffers.

Does this mean that, to maintain OA unity, individual OA members must sacrifice personal freedom of thought and give up every outside concern and activity? Of course not. As individuals, we are free to believe in, and work for, any cause we choose. The Tenth Tradition asks us to leave these issues outside when we walk through the doors of OA. Even the most worthy of other causes has no place in an OA meeting.

The OA recovery program is essential to each of us. Our very survival depends on it. Without it, many of us would soon be so thoroughly occupied with compulsive eating we would have little time or energy left to do anything else—including effectively supporting those other causes that mean so much to us. This is why we are careful to guard our Fellowship from even the slightest connection with outside issues.

Not honoring the Tenth Tradition often seems quite innocent, but it can have far-reaching consequences. This was the case when a newspaper columnist, syndicated around the world, stated in her advice column that a belief in Jesus Christ was an aspect of the OA program. Of course, OA has no opinion on Christianity or any other religion or spiritual belief, but the general public doesn't know this. Even after clarification from the World Service Office regarding this misrepresentation, the same perception was again carried in a subsequent column. The reason, according to a member of the columnist's staff, was that, despite our official disclaimer, the columnist had received letters over the years from compulsive overeaters who had been encouraged at OA meetings to "put their faith in Jesus Christ." Many suffering, nonreligious compulsive overeaters and those practicing other religions were no doubt needlessly discouraged from seeking OA's help because some members brought this outside issue into OA meetings.

Having no opinion on outside issues also means that we don't oppose any such causes. Ridicule and disrespectful comments about religions, diets, political beliefs, and other matters have absolutely no place in OA meetings. We don't need to belittle others in order to carry the message of recovery OA has to offer. In fact, negative talk and laughter at the expense of others usually interferes with the positive atmosphere of the OA meeting. Many of us suffer from the habit of negative thinking and speaking. We desperately need a positive atmosphere in our OA groups if we are to recover. Thus, we see the wisdom of keeping silent about outside issues in OA meetings.

What, exactly, are outside issues? This question has arisen more than once among us. For instance, many OA members are also members of other Twelve Step fellowships, and these groups sometimes have a place in the stories shared in OA meetings. OA as a whole, however, has no opinion on any group or treatment for alcoholism, drug use, codependency, or other compulsive disorders, and we find it best not to get sidetracked by them in OA meetings. Thus, OA groups focus their discussions on recovery from compulsive eating and compulsive food behaviors through OA's Twelve Steps and Twelve Traditions, rather than on these other issues.

But what about other programs and treatments for weight loss and eating disorders? These, too, are matters about which OA has no opinion. As individuals, we might share our experiences with them, but as an organization, we have nothing whatever to say either for or against any of them. We speak about the OA program in OA meetings. Our experience with it, honestly shared, never fails to offer hope and strength to the suffering compulsive overeater.

In honoring Tradition Ten, OA groups sell and display only OA-approved literature at their meetings and do not use outside literature as a basis for their group studies.[21] Many books and pamphlets have been written that are worthwhile and may have aided

---

[21] For many years, Alcoholics Anonymous books were the only books about the Steps and Traditions available, and they have been used extensively in OA groups. *Alcoholics Anonymous*, 4th ed. (Big Book), AA *Twelve Steps and Twelve Traditions*, and several other AA books are on the *OA-Approved Literature List* (© Overeaters Anonymous, Inc.). OA groups may stock these on their literature tables and read from them as part of their meeting formats.

individuals' recovery, but they have not been approved by OA as a whole. A policy of not using, selling, or displaying these publications in OA groups certainly isn't intended to ban their use among our membership. It simply means we have no opinion whatsoever on them. OA members' experience can be found in our own literature. Our books and pamphlets are developed, edited, and reviewed by committees made up of OA members from around the world. This doesn't mean, of course, that we all agree with everything in every OA publication. It simply means that they focus on OA Principles and the OA message of recovery from compulsive eating and compulsive food behaviors through the Twelve Steps of Overeaters Anonymous.

We compulsive eaters can learn a lot from OA's Tenth Tradition about concentrating on our message and avoiding controversy. It is summed up in the saying "live and let live." We find we can live happier and more effective lives when we focus our attention on doing our Higher Power's will each day rather than on conflicts.

### How do we uphold Tradition Ten?

*Do we ever give the impression that there is an "OA opinion" on diets? On diet clubs' weight-loss programs? On medical interventions for weight loss? On medications? On psychiatrists and therapists? On eating disorders treatment centers? On churches, religions, or spiritual beliefs? On nutrition? On food plans? On exercise? On sugar? On other Twelve Step groups?*

*Do we ridicule any of these or show them disrespect?*

*Can we share our personal experience concerning them without mentioning names or giving the impression we are stating OA's opinion?*

*In our meeting format and group practices, is our group careful not to imply that OA has an opinion on any of these?*

*In sharing at our meetings, do we try to help newcomers understand the Twelve Step program of OA better?*

*Do we find OA more interesting when there's a spark of controversy in the group? Do we ever bring up outside issues just to get people stirred up?*

*Are we afraid to speak in favor of the Tenth Tradition when we hear others linking OA to outside issues?*

*Do we ever use our close contact with OA friends to campaign for outside issues?*

*Can we continue to share OA fellowship—and even close friendship —with people who don't share our opinions? Do we concentrate on our common bonds, rather than on our differences?*

Tradition Ten frees us to concentrate on recovery from compulsive eating without the conflicts that seem to rage in the world around us. Many of us have been drawn to the excitement of conflict. Of course, no group or person can live completely free of conflict, but in OA we learn we can live, and even thrive, with a minimum of strife.

OA has excitement enough to offer, as we see hopeless compulsive overeaters recover through the miracle of the Twelve Steps. This could not happen if we allowed outside issues to turn our Fellowship into a platform for debate. For this reason, the Tenth Tradition of having no opinion on outside issues is one of our most carefully guarded practices in OA.

# TRADITION ELEVEN

Our public relations policy is based on attraction rather than promotion; we need always maintain personal anonymity at the level of press, radio, films, television, and other public media of communication.

---

*SPIRITUAL PRINCIPLE*

**ANONYMITY**

I n Overeaters Anonymous, we have found hope at last, a way out of the bondage of food, compulsive eating, and compulsive food behaviors. Filled with enthusiasm for the OA program, many of us want to tell everyone who might be eating compulsively about OA. Carrying the message, after all, is an important part of the Steps and the primary purpose of the OA Fellowship. The Eleventh Tradition gives us some guidelines for carrying OA's message, guidelines all OA members need to be aware of as we begin to share our program with those outside of OA.

We publicize OA without promoting it. We want people to know what OA is and how to find our meetings. Thus, we use public media of communication—websites, radio, television, print, videos, displays at health fairs,[22] social media in keeping with OA guidelines,[23] etc.—to provide factual information about our program. However, we do not promote OA with personal appeals, celebrity endorsements, or other such means of persuasion.

Use of the media in a nonprofessional way allows OA to attract those who are ready to take advantage of what we have to offer. Few of us who are now part of this Fellowship tried OA the first time we heard about it. We may have needed this recovery program then, but it took a while for some of us to decide to come and be willing to work the Steps. Until we were ready, nobody could have "sold" us this program. As it was with us, so it is with other people who may benefit from OA. We carry the message best when we share frankly what OA is and what our own experience has been. In respecting the Eleventh Tradition, we respect the right of others to choose OA for themselves.

This is the public relations policy for the OA Fellowship. We do everything we can to tell people what OA is, how it works, and where we meet. We don't publish "before and after" pictures of our members in the media. We don't promise quick weight loss or guarantee results. We don't have celebrities appearing in front of the public to talk about their success with our program and to invite others to join.

In fact, the Eleventh Tradition states that all individuals maintain their personal anonymity when speaking of their OA participation in any public medium of communication. In keeping the Eleventh Tradition, those of us who write books or are interviewed for a newspaper story or a radio or TV broadcast have two options. We can avoid calling ourselves OA members (even if we say we're compulsive eaters). Then we are free to use our full names or have

---

[22] Refer to Overeaters Anonymous, Inc. Business Conference Policy Manual, Continuing Effect Motions 2008b, 2008c, 2008d, and 2008e.

[23] Refer to Overeaters Anonymous, Inc. Business Conference Policy Manual, Continuing Effect Motion 2011a. Amended 2016.

our faces shown. Here, the emphasis is on the individual, and we are not connected publicly with the OA program.

Our other option is to identify ourselves as OA members. When we do this, we make sure our faces are not shown and our last names are not used. When we are careful to honor the Eleventh Tradition in this way, the emphasis remains on OA, rather than on us, as individuals.

In dealing with the media, we sometimes make the mistake of assuming that interviewers and photographers already know about OA's Tradition of anonymity. Many media professionals have only superficial knowledge about OA. It's up to us to explain the Eleventh Tradition and ask them to honor our anonymity through not showing our faces and either not using our full names or by using fictitious names. When we ourselves write about our OA membership for the news media or in books, we use our first name and last initial in our bylines.[24]

While Overeaters Anonymous has no opinion on outside issues, including social media, the delegates of the 2016 World Service Business Conference recommend that any OA member, group, or service body using social media for OA public information and public awareness maintain the personal anonymity of OA members.

Members of Overeaters Anonymous are anonymous. The Fellowship is not. Members of Overeaters Anonymous using social media are responsible for maintaining their own personal anonymity and respecting the anonymity of other OA members.[25]

It is no accident that the word "anonymous" is part of our name. Personal anonymity at the public level shows the world that we take this Tradition seriously, and that others can join us and be assured their membership will be kept private.

Some of us have protested, "I have nothing to hide. TV and so-

---

[24] For guidelines for dealing with the media, see the *Public Information Service Manual* (Overeaters Anonymous, Inc., © 1991 … 2017).

[25] Overeaters Anonymous, Inc. Business Conference Policy Manual, Continuing Effect Motion 2011a. Amended 2016.

cial media are visual, and newcomers will be attracted by my weight loss and my story. Besides, I don't care who knows I'm a member."

This may be true, but it ignores the fact that OA is a spiritual program. When one person assumes the role of an OA spokesperson, his or her action poses problems of a spiritual nature for the individual and the OA Fellowship. It poses problems for individuals because we have nothing of lasting spiritual value to gain—and perhaps much to lose—by publicizing our OA recovery. When we ignore the Eleventh Tradition, we set ourselves apart from other OA members in order to take on the role of spokesperson. Being a celebrity can be fun, but inevitably our star status isolates us. Then we have a hard time asking other OA members for help when we need it. Humility is one of the essential qualities we must develop in order to recover from compulsive eating. Maintaining our anonymity at the level of the public media is one way we practice humility. It's one way we let go of personal ambition in order to keep ourselves in fit spiritual condition.

Those who ignore our Eleventh Tradition cause damage to OA's spirit of fellowship, which is essential to our healing. Such breaks of anonymity may bring the OA name before the public, but they cause concern among OA members and misrepresent the OA Fellowship to the public by placing personalities before principles. They imply that one member's personal recovery or relapse is linked to OA's success or failure. The Eleventh Tradition helps ensure that we don't hurt the OA Fellowship in our misguided attempts to promote it.

OA's insistence on personal anonymity and refusal to promote our program through celebrity endorsements or other techniques of persuasion make it different from commercial programs. Through our OA experience, we learn that we don't need to promote ourselves and our views to other people. In the past, we feared we would not be appreciated or loved if we didn't tell others about our personal or professional accomplishments. Now, we let go of that fear and quietly do God's will.

## How do we practice the Eleventh Tradition?

*How does our group make its meeting place and time known to compulsive eaters who might want to attend?*

*How does our group inform the public—or support our service bodies in informing the public—about the OA program?*

*Is our OA recovery attractive enough to draw other compulsive eaters to OA?*

*Do we talk about OA so fanatically, or so often, that we make it unattractive to the people in our lives?*

*Are we careful to keep members' faces and names out of the story when we discuss OA with reporters or write about it ourselves?*

*Does our group or service body provide information about our Eleventh Tradition to the news media in our area? Do we ask them to keep all members anonymous in news stories about OA?*

*Are we careful to protect our personal anonymity and that of other OA members when using social media?*

*Are we willing to speak up for the Eleventh Tradition whenever we see it being ignored?*

"Attraction rather than promotion" is good for us and essential for the OA Fellowship. Our individual recovery, as well as group unity and effectiveness, depends on this unusual type of public relations. The Eleventh Tradition is based on faith in our program and in that Power greater than ourselves that guides compulsive eaters to our doors. All we have to do is let the facts about OA and its Principles be known. We can depend on our Higher Power and this program to attract those who can benefit by what OA has to offer. When we maintain our Tradition of anonymity, we ensure that Overeaters Anonymous remains a spiritual Fellowship, supporting all of us in our recovery.[26]

---

[26] For more information on the subject of anonymity, see *Anonymity: The Meaning and Applications of Traditions Eleven and Twelve* (Overeaters Anonymous, Inc., © 1983).

# TRADITION TWELVE

Anonymity is the spiritual foundation of all these Traditions, ever reminding us to place principles before personalities.

---

*SPIRITUAL PRINCIPLE*

**SPIRITUALITY**

Living by the Twelve Traditions of Overeaters Anonymous requires that we adopt attitudes that seem strange at first to many of us. For instance, we place the welfare of the OA group above our own desires. We give up our aspirations to govern our fellow members. We welcome to our meetings all people with a desire to stop eating compulsively, no matter what we think or feel about them. We give up our dependence on authorities and power structures, along with our ambitions to climb to the top of some imagined OA ladder. We cease all attempts to use OA to promote our favorite outside issues and enterprises. We pay our own way and quit expecting others to keep OA going without our help. We give up all aspirations to gain status as special OA members. We give up all ambitions that we might someday be acclaimed for our OA recovery or service.

Behind all these self-sacrificing attitudes is a single spiritual foundation, so important to our Fellowship, it is part of our name: anonymity. Without a strong foundation, no house will stand for long. It is essential that all of us understand and respect anonymity if OA is to survive and we are to find recovery here.

Our experience with the many aspects of anonymity starts when we walk in the door as OA newcomers. At that point, many of us don't want anyone to know we're coming to OA, anything about our relationship with food, and the problems it has caused us, or how we feel about ourselves. In OA we find a haven, a place to share our feelings and experiences with other human beings who also suffer from the disease of compulsive eating and compulsive food behaviors. When we all respect the anonymity of others, we can trust that nobody outside these rooms will know we're coming to OA unless we tell them. Because ours is a program of Principles, not personalities, we expect that what we share here won't be gossiped about or judged, inside or outside of OA.

Yet anonymity means a great deal more to us than just not gossiping. The quality of our recovery ultimately depends on understanding and practicing anonymity as a spiritual Principle.

Many of us come to OA carrying the excess baggage of shame and pride. We are ashamed that we've been unable to control our eating by ourselves, and yet we're too proud to admit that we need help with our eating and our lives. In order to recover, we have to let go of shame and pride and actively reach out to others for help. As we practice anonymity, we begin this process of letting go.

To be anonymous in OA means to be one among many, to accept ourselves as no better or worse than our fellows. This acceptance places us in a state of humility and enables us to become teachable. We find ourselves listening intently to people whose last names we don't know. They may be older or younger than we are, more or less successful by material standards or may come from entirely different backgrounds. We listen because we identify with them. We've learned that they may say something that can help our recovery.

We often go on a first-name basis in OA meetings, not because we're embarrassed about our OA membership, but because last names simply aren't important. OA members may be famous or unknown. We may have many accomplishments or few, a lot of money or little. As we practice our Tradition of anonymity, we affirm an important truth: In OA, we're all on equal footing—reduced to helplessness by our compulsive eating and compulsive food behaviors and freed to recover by practicing this miraculous program. Money, intelligence, and status made no difference in our becoming compulsive overeaters and they make no difference in our chances for recovery.

Anonymity is not the same thing as secrecy. As OA's pamphlet *The Tools of Recovery* says, "It is not a break of anonymity to use our full names within our group or OA service bodies."[27] When we fully identify ourselves, many of us have found it is easier to carry out our service work and to reach out to one another when we need help. While we make every effort to avoid gossip, we need to remember "it is not a break of anonymity to enlist Twelfth-Step help for group members in trouble, provided we are careful to refrain from discussing any specific personal information."[28] For example, we might enlist such help without breaking a person's anonymity by saying, "Have you talked to Mary lately? She may find a phone call helpful."

We need to remember, too, that not all members immediately let go of the gossip habit when we enter the doors of OA, and there may be newcomers present who are unfamiliar with our Traditions. Therefore, it is recommended to share in a general way during OA meetings and save the more intimate details for our sponsors or others we have learned to trust in OA. Those who have walked the Twelve Step path before us know the sacred trust of receiving personal inventories and the importance of anonymity. Many of us find that the unconditional acceptance and trust that springs from the practice of anonymity opens us to one another in ways we have

---

[27] *The Tools of Recovery* (Overeaters Anonymous, Inc., © 1981 … 2011) p. 6.
[28] Ibid. p. 6.

never experienced before.

When we keep the Twelfth Tradition, no one person or group of people is ever given special status in OA. Our leaders have no special honors; they're simply our trusted servants. When we applaud someone's weight loss or celebrate abstinence anniversaries in our meetings, it doesn't mean we are singling out these people for glory. It means we are rejoicing in a fellow compulsive overeater's recovery. The OA member abstaining from compulsive eating is no more important than the member in relapse. Newcomers and young people share equally with longtime members in our meetings. Some members are called on to speak in front of large OA groups, but this doesn't make them more important than anyone else in the Fellowship. After they share, they usually sit down with the crowd and listen to the next speaker. They want to learn all they can, and they never know whom their Higher Power might choose to teach them.

In OA, we learn that our recovery comes to us through the Principles of the program, not through personalities. We discover that we can learn from and work in harmony with people whose personalities we dislike, as long as we focus on OA Principles. Many of us have had the experience of hearing fellow members we disliked say things we found helpful to our recovery.

We have also had the experience of setting certain members on pedestals, only to have them climb down or fall off. Sometimes we've tried to build our program around one person we admired, a sponsor or a speaker. The day inevitably came when that person seemed to fail us in some way, and our own recovery felt threatened. It was then we learned the importance of placing Principles before personalities. We have found through years of experience that the Principles of OA are failure-proof. They are the solid foundation upon which we can construct meaningful lives.

Over the years, our Fellowship has learned how important it is to emphasize these life-saving Principles rather than personalities when planning conventions and other events. In the past, OA members who are well-known as authors, speakers, or eating disorders experts have been invited to speak at special events. The groups and service bodies advertised those names on flyers and in newsletters. In some cases, hundreds of suffering compulsive overeaters flocked to hear the speaker. There was a short-term benefit, but over time, problems arose. Some speakers were more interested in self-promotion than in the Principles of the program. Some took advantage of their status to promote their books and treatment programs. Some struggling members placed their trust in these individuals, rather than in the Principles of the program. In one case, reports of personal abuses arose. Because those sponsoring the events had used these well-known members as star attractions, they found it difficult to prevent the breaches of the Traditions.

After years of such difficulties, OA delegates to the World Service Business Conference voted to suggest that "individual groups and service bodies refrain from publishing the names or non-OA titles of speakers/leaders at OA functions in any informational materials (flyers, newsletters, etc.). OA service titles (but not names) may be used when a speaker/leader is performing the service responsibility of her or his OA office."[29]

Anonymity fosters humility and guards against reemergence of that blind self-will that leads back to compulsive eating. Prevented by our Traditions from placing ourselves or others in a position of distinction within our Fellowship, we find it easier for each of us simply to be a part of the group. This is essential to recovery from our disease of isolation. It means supporting and being supported by our fellow OA members and sharing openly the joys and challenges of our lives. These are things we could never afford to do in any group where we were trying to make names for ourselves.

Thus, it is to promote our own recovery that we cultivate the attitude of humility implied in Tradition Twelve. As we continue to grow spiritually, we begin to lose our desire for prestige in OA and in other areas of our lives. It is satisfaction enough to be in recovery—fully functioning and contributing as human beings. And we know we can't take all the credit even for that. We share credit with

---

[29] Overeaters Anonymous, Inc. Business Conference Policy Manual, Continuing Effect Motion 1990. Amended 2011 and 2014.

our Higher Power and our fellow OA members who have supported us and taught us so much. We also accept responsibility for our actions, looking only at our own faults and taking no one's inventory but our own.

**In what ways do we act "to place principles before personalities"?**

*Does our group always inform newcomers and remind all who attend about the meaning and importance of anonymity in OA?*

*Are we careful not to mention OA members' names to impress others, even within the Fellowship?*

*Do we ever repeat anything personal we have heard at meetings or from other members?*

*Do we value all OA members equally, or do we give some individuals special status?*

*Does our group support and trust our group conscience, or do we let one, or several, strong personalities run things?*

*Do we speak up for OA Principles, no matter who might be displeased?*

*Do we ever confuse OA Principles with our personal opinions?*

*Do we make our full identity known within the group so we can be called on for Twelfth Step work?*

*Are we ever tempted to look at our OA "success" as a way to gain personal recognition?*

As we recover in OA, we come to feel that anonymity is one of our most precious possessions. Anonymity is the spiritual foundation of our transformed lives, as well as of OA's Traditions. We are compulsive eaters, living in recovery, no longer in bondage to food. We know that support for our recovery will always be here for us, as long as we remember "to place principles before personalities," respecting these vital Twelve Traditions that bind us together in the Fellowship of Overeaters Anonymous.

# THE TWELVE STEPS of Overeaters Anonymous

1. We admitted we were powerless over food—that our lives had become unmanageable.

2. Came to believe that a power greater than ourselves could restore us to sanity.

3. Made a decision to turn our will and our lives over to the care of God *as we understood Him.*

4. Made a searching and fearless moral inventory of ourselves.

5. Admitted to God, to ourselves, and to another human being the exact nature of our wrongs.

6. Were entirely ready to have God remove all these defects of character.

7. Humbly asked Him to remove our shortcomings.

8. Made a list of all persons we had harmed and became willing to make amends to them all.

9. Made direct amends to such people wherever possible, except when to do so would injure them or others.

10. Continued to take personal inventory and when we were wrong, promptly admitted it.

11. Sought through prayer and meditation to improve our conscious contact with God *as we understood Him,* praying only for knowledge of His will for us and the power to carry that out.

12. Having had a spiritual awakening as the result of these Steps, we tried to carry this message to compulsive overeaters and to practice these principles in all our affairs.

*Permission to use the Twelve Steps of Alcoholics Anonymous for adaptation granted by AA World Services, Inc.*

1. Our common welfare should come first; personal recovery depends upon OA unity.

2. For our group purpose there is but one ultimate authority—a loving God as He may express Himself in our group conscience. Our leaders are but trusted servants; they do not govern.

3. The only requirement for OA membership is a desire to stop eating compulsively.

4. Each group should be autonomous except in matters affecting other groups or OA as a whole.

5. Each group has but one primary purpose—to carry its message to the compulsive overeater who still suffers.

6. An OA group ought never endorse, finance, or lend the OA name to any related facility or outside enterprise, lest problems of money, property, and prestige divert us from our primary purpose.

7. Every OA group ought to be fully self-supporting, declining outside contributions.

8. Overeaters Anonymous should remain forever nonprofessional, but our service centers may employ special workers.

9. OA, as such, ought never be organized; but we may create service boards or committees directly responsible to those they serve.

10. Overeaters Anonymous has no opinion on outside issues; hence the OA name ought never be drawn into public controversy.

11. Our public relations policy is based on attraction rather than promotion; we need always maintain personal anonymity at the level of press, radio, films, television, and other public media of communication.

12. Anonymity is the spiritual foundation of all these Traditions, ever reminding us to place principles before personalities.

*Permission to use the Twelve Traditions of Alcoholics Anonymous for adaptation granted by AA World Services, Inc.*

For more information on
Overeaters Anonymous,
write to the
World Service Office
PO Box 44020
Rio Rancho, NM 87174-4020 USA
or email info@oa.org.
www.oa.org

# INDEX

## A

abstinence, 4, 18, 19, 83, 101, 116
  anniversaries of, 82, 166
  definition of, 20
  maintaining, 20, 21, 57, 108, 109
  opinions on achieving, 108
  problems with, 43, 109
  recovery and, 43, 57
  responsibility for, 143

abuse, 12, 30, 31, 35, 43, 117, 167

acceptance
  love and, 13, 95
  unconditional, 41, 43, 72, 75, 112,
    165

action, 42, 63, 66, 73
  amends for, 67
  group, 113, 114
  on-the-spot, 71
  patterns and, 70
  taking, 80
  willingness for, 45-46

action plan, 21

Alcoholics Anonymous, 89

*Alcoholics Anonymous, Fourth
Edition,* 28, 54
  *See also* Big Book

amends
  anonymous, 67
  appropriateness of, 66-67
  change and, 65-66
  direct/indirect, 66
  forgiveness and, 62
  living, 66
  making, 57-62, 63-67, 71, 73
  recovery and, 62

anger, 5, 6, 25, 30, 65, 105

anonymity, 21, 67, 115, 121, 150
  humility and, 167
  maintaining, 157-61, 164
  practicing, 164, 165
  recovery and, 167

  service and, 150
  as spiritual foundation, 163-68
  tradition of, 159

anorexia, 1, 110, 117

anxieties, 6, 11, 31

apologies, 64, 65, 66

attitude, 25
  change in, 18, 79, 83-84
  harmful, 66

authority, 29, 99-105
  avoiding, 147
  dependence on, 163

autonomy, 110, 121
  group, 113-18
  principle of, 116, 118
  responsibility and, 113

awareness, 52, 43, 72
  spiritual, 67, 75-80, 81-87, 120

## B

behavior, 28, 29, 34-35, 148
  acknowledging, 40-41
  changing, 47, 49, 55
  compulsive food, 1, 4, 5-6, 19, 20,
    26, 57, 157, 108, 164
  destructive, 7, 27, 45, 46, 48, 56, 60,
    64, 66
  patterns of, 73
  reviewing, 25, 71, 74

belittling, 32, 41, 65, 93, 96, 153

Big Book, 28, 117, 142

binge eating, 1, 108, 136

Board of Trustees (OA), 116

body image, obsession with, 5, 91

bulimia, 1, 110, 117

## C

challenges, 49, 67, 75, 76, 82, 85, 99, 121
  facing, 44, 89-90, 167

change, 13, 15, 52, 73, 83-84
  amends and, 65-66
  fear of, 48
  need for, 12
  recovery and, 26-27, 41, 102
  undertaking, 65
  willingness for, 47, 48-49, 55, 64

character, 3, 28, 36, 47, 72
  shortcomings and, 55

character defects, 27
  awareness of, 43
  comfort from, 48
  Higher Power and, 45-49, 71, 72
  impact of, 46, 58
  insights into, 54
  rationalizing, 46-47
  removing, 44, 45, 46, 47, 48, 53, 56,
    72, 73, 74
  written inventory of, 54

cheating, 33, 35

committees, 102, 104, 139, 145-50

common welfare, attention to, 91-97

communication, 96, 157-58

compassion, spirit of, 139

compulsive eating, 1
  abstaining from, 6, 18, 20, 108
  confining, 11
  consequences of, 52
  desire to stop, 107-12, 163,164
  disease of, 4, 107
  emotional/physical/spiritual
    nature of, 5
  pain of, 108, 120
  return of, 5, 10, 11, 21

conflict, 147, 148, 155
  perpetuating, 29

control, 28
  losing, 5, 10
  manipulation and, 104

controversies, avoiding, 151-55

courage, 25-37, 85, 120

cravings, 4, 9

## D

decision making, 18, 102
  group conscience, 101, 118
  Higher Power and, 22-23
  influencing, 132
  informed, 100
  participation in, 134-35

denial, 5, 7, 26, 33, 70

depression, 5, 12

diet clubs, 10, 154

diets, 1, 5, 18, 19, 154
  compulsive, 94
  obsessing over, 10

disagreements, resolving, 29, 93, 94-96,
  111, 114

dishonesty, 13, 25, 26, 28, 33, 47, 55,
  65, 72

disrespect, 153, 154

diversity, 92
  embracing, 96, 110

drug use, 153

## E

eating
  controlling, 3
  guidelines, 4, 21
  obsession with, 91
  self-destructive, 58, 70
  uncontrolled, 4-5

embarrassment, 40, 59, 65, 67, 165

emotional balance, 4, 70, 83, 97

emotions, 37, 44, 82, 115
  awareness of, 72
  clarifying, 61
  reviewing, 71

events, organizing, 118, 131, 134, 146

experiences, 95, 101, 141
  sharing, 92, 127, 139, 140, 143, 153

**F**

faith, 17-23, 72, 85, 120

false pride, 32

fasting, 10, 108

faults, 12
  acknowledging, 63, 168

fear, 6, 11, 25, 31, 43, 46, 72, 136
  removing, 55

feelings, 46
  amends for, 67
  negative, 42, 60, 61, 71
  writing down, 61, 71, 78

fellowship, 56, 121, 131, 139-43, 155, 161
  common welfare of, 92
  emphasis on, 146
  group conscience and, 147
  joining, 39-40, 168
  spirit of, 160

financial support, responsibility for, 131-37

First Tradition Committee, 93

food
  causing compulsive eating, 19
  obsession with, 11, 18-19
  powerlessness over, 3-7
  problem with, 108
  restricting, 4
  thinking about, 18-19, 37

food plans, compulsive, 84

*For Today,* 69

forgiveness, 64
  amends and, 62
  healing and, 58, 59
  importance of, 60-61
  reconciliation and, 60

freedom of thought, 152

friendships, 155
  conditions on, 111
  controlling, 104
  developing, 40, 121
  experiencing, 12-13
  *See also* relationships

**G**

God. *See* Higher Power

gossiping, 33, 46, 96, 164

gratification, 29, 53, 83

group conscience, 92, 109, 132, 149, 169
  decision making and, 118
  discussions, 102, 104
  expressing, 103
  fellowship and, 147
  Higher Power and, 104
  informed, 100, 114
  leadership and, 102
  majority rule and, 100
  voting and, 101, 104

groups, primary purpose of, 117, 119-23

grudges, holding, 30, 42, 64

guilt, 28, 36, 40, 58, 60, 64, 65, 72
  feeling, 34
  unresolved, 26

**H**

harm, 72
  making amends for, 57-62, 63-67

healing, 15, 69
  emotional, 25
  forgiveness and, 59
  freedom and, 67
  writing and, 60-61

healing power, 120, 142, 148

Higher Power
  admitting wrongs to, 39-44, 70
  authority of, 99-105
  belief in, 12, 13, 14, 27, 67, 161
  change and, 47, 49, 52
  character defects and, 45-49, 71, 72
  conscious contact with, 75-80
  dependence on, 21, 161
  group conscience and, 104
  guidance from, 13, 18, 19, 20, 21, 42, 55, 73, 78, 99, 135, 136, 147, 149
  healing power of, 14, 53
  help from, 9-16, 18, 21, 22-23, 56, 73, 80
  knowledge of, 77-78

listening to, 79, 80, 101
love and, 13, 53
prayer and, 77, 78
recovery and, 14-15
relationship with, 15, 20, 75-76, 77, 78-79
shortcomings and, 51-56
trust in, 22, 43, 48, 53, 82, 85, 93, 103, 114, 136, 149, 150
turning lives over to, 14-15, 17-23, 19, 23, 70, 74, 78, 84
will of, 23, 80, 99, 105, 154

honesty, 3-7, 11, 20, 40, 41, 84-86, 96, 120, 139
attitudes about, 74
importance of, 44
increase in, 26
looking with, 9
relationships and, 59, 72

hope, 9-15, 86, 95, 120
sharing, 92, 139, 143

humiliation, 41, 51, 52, 59

humility, 44, 51-56, 120, 142, 149, 150, 160, 164
achieving, 51, 53-54, 167
anonymity and, 167
recovery and, 53

hurt, 61, 85
making amends and, 63-67

## I

identity, 107-12

integrity, 39-44, 85, 120

intergroups, 93-94, 100, 123, 131, 132, 146
decision making by, 134-35
financial support for, 133, 134
representatives to, 137
special workers for, 140

intimidation, 28, 35

isolation, 31, 39, 40, 70, 86, 91, 101, 148

## J

jealousy, 28, 30, 42

## L

leadership
group conscience and, 102
professional, 142
reimbursing, 141
as trusted servants, 99, 166

*Lifeline,* 117, 121, 132, 147

literature, 21, 27, 77, 80, 115, 122, 127, 129, 131, 132
OA-approved, 126, 148
publishing, 102-3

love, 56, 63-67, 75, 120
acceptance and, 13, 95
healing power of, 1, 53
self-discipline and, 85-86

lying, 9-10, 46

## M

manipulation, 28, 35, 104

media, 157-58, 159, 160
nonprofessional use of, 158

meditation, 36, 55, 117
contact with God and, 75-80

meetings, 12, 13, 21, 39, 40, 76, 77, 80, 84, 92, 94, 96, 118
attending, 75, 89
autonomy of, 110
harmony of, 109
special-focus, 110, 117

membership
group, 116, 117
guidelines for, 116
privacy in, 159-60
requirement of, 107-12

message
carrying, 87, 119-23, 129, 148, 153, 157-58
focus on, 154

mistakes, 63, 114, 147
admitting, 33, 65, 72, 85

moral inventory, 40, 54, 168
recovery and, 27, 36-37
searching and fearless, 25-37

taking, 26, 28, 69-74
writing, 26, 27, 36, 58

motives, 72, 79
understanding, 42-43

## N

neutrality, 121, 151-55

newcomers, 118, 139, 154, 166
speaking to, 111, 121, 122

nonorganization, tradition of, 147

nonprofessionalism
practicing, 142-43
tradition of, 139-43

nutrition, 10, 19, 20, 154

## O

obesity, avoiding, 5

obsession, 5, 10, 11, 18-19, 52, 57, 91
freedom from, 18, 21, 23
with money, 29
relieving, 17, 21

office management, hiring, 140, 141

opinions, 154
differences in, 93, 107, 151

organization, 147
freedom from, 145, 146

outside contributions, 131-37

outside enterprises, 125-29, 163
endorsement from, 126-27

outside issues, opinion on, 151-55

overeating, 1, 9, 11

overexercising, 1, 5

## P

pain, 61, 74

participation, 109, 128

perfectionism, 21, 26, 27, 29, 47

perseverance, 69-74, 86

personal problems, 109, 122

personalities
conflicting, 115
principles and, 168

plan of eating, a, 20, 21, 26, 94, 95

Power greater than ourselves. *See* Higher Power

power structures, 100, 163

powerlessness, 3-7, 81, 84-85
admission of, 6-7, 10, 17, 26

prayer, 14, 23, 53, 54, 72
contact with God and, 75-80
daily, 55, 61, 76-77
experiencing, 79-80
Higher Power and, 78
spiritual connection with, 86
trying, 61, 79
for willingness, 27

pride, 25, 32-33, 164

primary purpose, 157
diversion from, 125-29

Principles, 92, 95
living by, 1, 13, 53, 115, 120-21
personalities and, 168
practicing, 115, 120, 121
recovery and, 145, 166
*See also* spiritual Principles

problem solving, 11, 42, 103, 119

problems, 69
coping with, 82
emotional/spiritual nature of, 18
sharing, 142

procrastination, 6, 27, 29, 63

psychology, 74, 141, 142

public relations policy, 157-61

publications, 84, 131, 132, 146, 152, 153, 167
financing, 134
non-OA-approved, 126
OA-approved, 126

purging, 1, 4, 5, 10, 108

purpose, 119-23

**R**

rationalization, 40, 79

recovery, 1, 59, 61, 64, 70, 75-76, 84, 101, 108, 109, 117, 139, 147, 165, 166, 167-68
  abstinence and, 43, 57
  amends and, 62
  anniversaries of, 82
  anonymity and, 167
  approaches to, 92, 93, 95
  attractiveness of, 161
  beginning, 3, 7, 23
  change and, 26-27, 41, 102
  companions in, 83
  continuing toward, 36
  delaying, 26-27, 47, 109, 111
  finding, 12, 13, 84, 92, 94, 114
  focus on, 89, 115, 122, 125-29, 132, 140, 152, 153, 155
  healing power and, 120
  helping with, 128, 165
  Higher Power and, 14-15
  humility and, 53
  inventory and, 27, 36-37
  message of, 89, 119, 120, 123, 134, 141, 145, 153, 154
  need for, 121, 158
  permanent, 69, 74, 86, 164
  public relations and, 161
  responsibility and, 119, 143
  sharing, 114, 123
  spiritual program and, 119
  support for, 151, 161
  therapy groups and, 142
  unity and, 91-97
  willingness and, 55

region, 93, 94, 97, 122, 123, 132, 137
  support for, 133, 134

relationships
  abusive, 11-12, 31
  controlling, 104
  damaging, 10, 30, 63
  developing, 13, 40, 57, 64, 66, 67, 86, 132
  eating behaviors and, 5-6
  honesty and, 59, 72
  improving, 57, 64, 66, 67

religious beliefs, 12, 13, 77, 152

resentment, 25, 30, 40, 72, 74, 78
  removing, 55, 61

responsibility, 20, 29-30, 92, 101, 103, 121, 122, 131-37
  autonomy and, 113
  recovery and, 119
  taking, 35, 102, 118, 129, 148, 149, 168

restitution, making, 63-67

**S**

sanity, 9-15, 17, 19, 21

secrets, 25, 87
  hidden, 34, 41, 43

security, 30, 102

self-analysis, 26, 28, 71

self-awareness, 26, 73

self-centeredness, 6, 25, 28-30, 32

self-destruction, 9, 55, 82

self-discipline, 57-62, 120
  love and, 85-86

self-esteem, 34, 51, 53, 56
  loss of, 10, 30, 48, 52, 67

self-examination, 11, 26

self-forgiveness, 42-43, 51, 60

self-knowledge, nutrition and, 20

self-righteousness, 30, 52

self-supporting, importance of being, 115, 131-37

self-will, 23, 71, 167

serenity, 57, 61, 71

Serenity Prayer, 94

service, 21, 81-87, 89, 100, 101, 102, 104, 108, 120, 123, 135, 137, 139, 140, 141, 142, 146, 149, 164, 165
  anonymity and, 150
  humility and, 150
  opportunity for, 92
  spirit of, 143

service boards, 100, 123, 131, 137
  creating, 145-50
  decision making by, 134-35
  supporting, 122

service bodies, 83, 102, 104, 122, 137, 149, 167
  financial support for, 133, 134, 136
  Twelve Traditions and, 89

service centers, special workers for, 139-43

service work, 100, 102, 134, 135, 137, 139

sexual attitudes, 25, 34-35

shame, 34, 40, 164

sharing, 96, 122, 129, 148, 149, 167
  depth of, 139
  guidelines for, 116
  spirit of, 142

shortcomings, 41, 43
  accepting, 36, 54
  character traits and, 55
  removing, 47, 51-56, 85

sincerity, 22, 23, 36, 55, 60, 61, 65, 80

social lives, denying, 10

social media, 159-60, 161

solidarity, 121, 125-29

speaking, 96, 100, 141, 153, 167

special events, 122, 146

special workers, employing, 139-43

spiritual awareness, 75-80

spiritual growth, 18, 49, 76, 77, 79, 82, 89, 97, 164
  helping with, 128
  journey of, 86
  openness to, 12
  path of, 84

spiritual power, idea of, 13

spiritual Principles
  Step One, Honesty, 3-7
  Step Two, Hope, 9-15
  Step Three, Faith, 17-23
  Step Four, Courage, 25-37
  Step Five, Integrity, 39-44
  Step Six, Willingness, 45-49
  Step Seven, Humility, 51-56
  Step Eight, Self-Discipline, 57-62
  Step Nine, Love, 63-67
  Step Ten, Perseverance, 69-74
  Step Eleven, Spiritual Awareness, 75-80
  Step Twelve, Service, 81-87
  Tradition One, Unity, 91-97
  Tradition Two, Trust, 99-105
  Tradition Three, Identity, 107-12
  Tradition Four, Autonomy, 113-18
  Tradition Five, Purpose, 119-23
  Tradition Six, Solidarity, 125-29
  Tradition Seven, Responsibility, 131-37
  Tradition Eight, Fellowship, 139-43
  Tradition Nine, Structure, 145-50
  Tradition Ten, Neutrality, 151-55
  Tradition Eleven, Anonymity, 157-61
  Tradition Twelve, Spirituality, 163-68
  See also Principles

spirituality, 12, 121, 142, 152, 154, 160, 163-68
  recovery and, 119

sponsors, 13, 42, 64, 71, 72, 80, 139, 142, 167
  discussions with, 92
  finding, 123
  willingness and, 59

sponsorship, 21, 97

Step One, 3-7

Step Two, 9-15

Step Three, 17-23

Step Four, 25-37, 54

Step Five, 39-44

Step Six, 45-49

Step Seven, 51-56
  Prayer, 54

Step Eight, 57-62

Step Nine, 63-67

Step Ten, 69-74

Step Eleven, 75-80
Step Twelve, 81-87
strength, 95
    sharing, 92, 139, 143
structure, 121, 145-50
stubbornness, 56, 70

**T**

telephone, 21, 40, 83, 96, 123, 125, 126, 165
therapy groups, 84, 127, 141-42
thinking, 42
    changing, 47, 49
    destructive, 46, 48, 58
    failed, 7
    focusing on, 28
    negative, 25, 27, 33-34, 153
    positive, 73
    writing down, 71
Tools of recovery, listed, 21
*Tools of Recovery, The,* 165
Tradition One, 91-97, 100
    practicing, 95-96
Tradition Two, 99-105
    practicing, 104-5
Tradition Three, 107-12
    practicing, 111-12
Tradition Four, 113-18
    practicing, 117-18
Tradition Five, 115, 119-23, 133
    practicing, 123
Tradition Six, 115, 125-29, 126
    practicing, 129
Tradition Seven, 115, 131-37
    practicing, 136-37
Tradition Eight, 132, 139-43
    practicing, 142-43
Tradition Nine, 145-50
    practicing, 149-50
Tradition Ten, 115, 151-55

practicing, 152, 154-55
Tradition Eleven, 157-61
    practicing, 159, 161
Tradition Twelve, 163-68
    practicing, 168
treatment programs, 125, 126-27, 129, 167
    sharing about, 127
trust, 31, 43, 44, 99-105, 120
    unconditional, 165
truth, 10, 86
    acknowledging, 7, 40-41
*Twelve-Step Workbook of Overeaters Anonymous, The,* 27
*Twelve Step Workshop and Study Guide,* 28
Twelve Steps, 1
    commitment to, 100, 140, 148
    listed, 169
    working, 15, 19, 21, 22, 23, 36, 53, 74, 108, 116, 146, 168
Twelve Traditions
    commitment to, 140
    listed, 170
    living by, 1, 100, 101, 108, 115, 146
    meetings/service bodies and, 89

**U**

unity
    disagreements and, 93, 94-96
    maintaining, 92, 120, 152
    practicing, 95-96
    public relations policy and, 161
    recovery and, 91-97
    truth of, 97
Unity Day celebrations, 94
"Unity with Diversity" Policy, 110

**V**

voting, 100, 116, 146, 149
    group conscience, 101, 104

# W

weight loss, 5, 10, 18
  celebrating, 94, 166
  programs, 18, 153, 154

willingness, 45-49, 54, 59-60, 85, 120
  for change, 47, 48-49, 55, 64
  prayer for, 27
  for taking action, 45-46

willpower, 3-4, 12, 23, 34

World Service Business Conference,
  103, 109, 135, 137, 159, 167

World Service Office, 108, 110, 114,
  115, 123, 132, 137, 146
  Board of Trustees and, 116
  financial support for, 122, 133, 134,
    136
  misrepresentations and, 152

writing, 21, 26, 27, 28, 36, 54, 58, 59,
  66, 71, 73, 78, 83
  healing and, 60-61

wrongs, admitting, 39-44, 66, 69-74